SHARED HUMANITY

A FIELD AGENT'S JOURNEY INTO THE HUMAN MIND

ROBERT GILLESPIE, PHD

GENERATIONAL COPY LLC

Cover design by David Ter-Avanesyan/Ter33Design LLC

ISBN: 979-8-9884350-6-8

Publisher: Generational Copy LLC

Published in the United States of America

SHARED HUMANITY

A FIELD AGENT'S JOURNEY INTO THE HUMAN MIND

ROBERT GILLESPIE, PHD

CONTENTS

AUTHOR'S NOTE

The story of my paternal grandfather running away from home to become a seafarer has always intrigued me.

As explained by my father, my grandfather was the first generation of his Irish American family to be born in America, but when he was 16, his parents, who had done well financially in the Irish linen trade during the 1870s, sent him to a private Jesuit seminary in upstate New York to civilize him.

Rebelling against the monkish restrictions of the school, in the dead of night, he and a cousin leapt from a window making their way to the docks of New York to stow themselves away on a sailing ship. When they were finally discovered, the ship was already out to sea, and the captain, having no real use for them, made them cabin boys to assist the officers with their daily chores. However, when his cousin found himself at odds with the captain, both boys decided to jump ship in Rio de Janeiro.

After living on the beach for six months, the two young men, now in rags, stowed away on another sailing ship bound for New York. Unlike their last trip, when they were discovered, the ship's captain saw some promise and offered to train them as merchant seaman, which appealed to my grandfather. They worked their way from city to city transporting passengers and cargo, but when the ship encountered a turbulent storm that nearly killed them, he decided that the life of a seamen was not for him. His cousin, however, continued to follow the ocean's call for the rest of his life.

Despite being on land again, my grandfather continued to feel a sense of wanderlust and eventually decided to take a job with the Pennsylvania Railroad, which bore routes through the northeastern United States up to Canada, as far west as St. Louis and Chicago, and as far south as Washington, D.C. and Virginia. He spent several years working as a roustabout[1] traveling around the country until one day, in a boarding house in small town in Pennsylvania, he fell in love with the daughter of the boarding house's owner. When my grandfather asked for her hand in marriage, her father, who was himself a retired train conductor, refused to bless the union unless my grandfather gave up his wandering ways. Acquiescing, he quit his job with the railroad, returned to his family in New York, found what his fiancée's father termed "stable and respectable work", and settled down with his new bride to start a family.

My father told me that when my grandfather would reminisce about the adventures of his youth, a distant expression would appear in his eyes as if he were again navigating the seas or wandering the countryside.

Like him, I have been a wanderer all my life; however, while my grandfather adventured into the vast terra incognito fleeing the confinement of the seminary, I've navigated the unchartered archipelago of the human psyche in pursuit of our shared humanity.

In this quest, I became a psychologist and psychotherapist, traveling far from my parochial Irish Catholic roots on the edge

---

1.   A roustabout on the railroad refers to a laborer or worker who performs various manual tasks.

of the megalopolis of New York City. While the road I've followed has had many twists and sometimes been as treacherous as the seas my grandfather sailed, the people I encountered along the way have confirmed for me a postulate from the famous psychiatrist Harry Stack Sullivan:

"We are all much more simply human than otherwise..."

This story takes place in a variety of clinical settings ranging from large trauma centers and rehabilitation hospitals to private consulting offices. It spans the continent north to south and east to west, from New York City and Connecticut to Florida, Northern California, and the Midwest. It is, however, not a travelogue. While the events that take place are set against the backdrop of my own transition from working as a government field agent to finally becoming a psychotherapist, the primary focus is on my patients' struggles as we both engage in the human enterprise of psychotherapy.

In sharing these stories, I have taken care to protect my patients' anonymity by changing their names and other identifying details while retaining the essence of their experience in the most authentic form possible. I have not changed the names of most of the colleagues and mentors in hopes that they will recognize the love and immense respect that I have for them.

While these stories reflect how the practice of psychology and neuropsychology shaped my clinical thinking, the purpose of this book is neither to showcase my career accolades and achievements nor to present my patients' lives and struggles from a purely scientific lens as if they were test subjects in a lab. Rather, my hope is that this book conveys the shared humanity of my patients in a way that reflects their complex lives in the most compassionate and respectful way possible. If in any way this does not come through, please know that it was never my aim or intention.

Lastly, I want to clarify that this is not a technical manual or a how-to guide on psychotherapy. It is, rather, an intimate glimpse into the mind and experiences of both therapist and patient as we work together. At times, the information I share may feel technical and scientific, but my goal is that you feel as if you were sitting beside me engaging in the practice of psychotherapy.

I dedicate this book to my extraordinary wife, Astrid, who has been my lifelong compadre and consigliere. She has faithfully participated with me in every single adventure in this book. I also dedicate this book to my sons, Robert and Richard, for their patient and persistent interest in their 'old man's' stories. Their love, ideas, and support have been crucial in helping me to create this work. Also, my thanks to my grandson, Luke, for his ideas regarding the title of this work.

Finally, I would like to thank my editor, Knikki Hernandez, for her wonderful insights and comments on this work. Without her technical and creative expertise, this project would never have come to completion.

Dr. G
Davenport, Iowa
2025

My reasons for the journey
The details are obscure
But I do believe
It was a holy grail
That I was looking for.

Dr. G, 2021

PROLOGUE: ORIGINS

Alcohol Research Center Laboratory
University of Connecticut Medical Center
West Hartford, 1984

THERE IT IS! That sensation. I feel it again before I can give it a name.

In the darkened monitoring room of a laboratory deep in the bowels of the university medical center, a tightness in my chest begins to swell. It's accompanied by an increase in my heart and respiration rate, which reminds me of how similar these sensations are to anxiety, but this is not that. This is the exhilaration of discovery that sits on the razor's edge between excitement and fear.

I have experienced this feeling before as a government investigator. It is the aha! moment in an investigation when all the pieces of the puzzle suddenly take shape and fall into a recognizable pattern. What makes this particular discovery so momentous is that the data we're collecting contradicts the *pensée du jour*[1] on the subject of addiction, revealing what drives human behavior at the unconscious level.

I'm at the end of my doctoral training in clinical psychology and am a member of a scientific research team at the University of Connecticut's Alcohol Research Center (ARC) studying the reasons behind high relapse rates for patients who have undergone intensive inpatient treatment for addiction. Current numbers reflect a 50-60% relapse rate within the first three months after discharge[2] and a 93% rate within the first five years after treatment[3]. The experiment, which will be the basis of my dissertation, is designed to explore this phenomenon.

The patient on the other side of the lab's one-way glass is dressed in hospital pajamas and suffers from alcoholism. At the end of his inpatient treatment program, he has volunteered to participate in this experiment. He's been abstinent from alcohol for four weeks and wants to do everything in his power to remain sober.

His body is connected to various devices that record an array of involuntary physiological responses including his heart, respiratory, and perspiration rate as well as his temperature. Any moment now, he is about to be exposed to his

---

1. *Pensée du jour — thought of the day.* In this context the prevailing theories of the day.
2. Hunt, Barnett & Branch, 1971
3. Emerick & Hansen, 1983

favorite type of alcohol so we can assess the changes in his physiology and cravings.

The most current explanation for relapse is the cognitive-behavioral model[4]. While there has been intense debate between the role of early development as the basis for addictive behaviors in adulthood, cognitive behaviorism[5] is now the dominate model we use to treat patients.

Based on this theory, thoughts control feelings, and feelings drive behaviors. For patients who are in high-risk situations where alcohol may be present, many experience shifts in their thought patterns, moving from *I will maintain my sobriety,* to *It would be nice to get high,* to *I want a drink,* which ultimately leads to relapse. The emphasis in this model is that the role of the individual's dysfunctional thinking causes their relapse.

Yet, what I've been observing in the lab over the past year is not consistent with this theory.

As we expected, the experimental alcoholic group, despite a verbalized commitment to remain abstinent, are experiencing a heightened craving for alcohol when exposed to their favorite beverages. However, what we didn't expect was that *before* their cravings began, the monitors showed several physiological responses such as increased sweating, heart rate, and salivation (a consummatory response[6]) that were not exhibited by the nonalcoholic control group. These responses, based on their self-reports, were all beneath their conscious awareness and significantly correlated with the evolution of their

---

4. The most popular treatment model Alcoholics Anonymous (AA) is atheoretical, psychoanalytic explanations have fallen out of favor as too vague and conditioning models (classical and operant) have been subsumed under the cognitive behavioral model.
5. A branch of psychology that emphasizes that behavior, thoughts, and feelings are all interrelated.
6. A consummatory response is an involuntary reflex or behavioral action taken to prepare for or fulfill a need.

thought patterns around alcohol. These are involuntary changes and originate in a primitive part of the brain known as the paleomammalian cortex[7], which regulates basic biological mechanisms for survival and operates largely outside of one's awareness or control.

This data strongly suggests that alcohol for these patients activates the paleomammalian cortex. Contrary to the cognitive behavioral model, this means that relapse isn't the result of the patients' maladaptive thinking patterns but rather *the unconscious physiological responses they experience in the presence of alcohol that affect their thoughts, feelings, and, subsequently, their behavior.* Put simply, the patients are not *thinking* themselves into relapse. They are being driven to it by a primitive neurological reaction—a response that we did not observe in the nonalcoholic subjects.

This finding is significant because it shows that there's an unaddressed vulnerability in treatment programs, which has far-teaching implications for for other psychological problems such as addiction, anxiety, trauma, and brain injury that involve the paleomammalian cortex.

As my gaze alternates between the experimental subject and the flashing lights of the recording devices, I see an image of myself dressed in a white lab coat reflected dimly in the one-way mirror. Staring at my reflection, the exhilaration bubbling within me is tempered by a strange thought: *Is this really me? A researcher dressed in a lab coat conducting an experiment? I was*

---

7. The paleomammalian cortex is a set of neurological structures involved in emotional processing and motivation in humans and other mammals. It is considered an evolutionarily older part of the brain primarily involved in the regulation of more primitive brain functions related to biological survival and procreation. It is in turn regulated by the evolutionarily younger and significantly more massive neocortex, which is the seat of conscious thought, logical reasoning, planning and language.

trained to work the streets, not a lab. As I look at my reflection, a disturbing memory of the fateful events that occurred in New York City nearly a decade ago emerges in my mind—the consequences of which, had they not have happened at all, would have altered the trajectory of my life, and I might not have become a psychologist or been in this lab at all.

~

Manhattan College
New York City, 1969

The warmth of summer is just heating up. As I recline with my girlfriend on a blanket upon the manicured lawn of the college quad, music from a concert by the folk artist Arlo Guthrie fills the air. He has just finished singing his antiwar song "Alice's Restaurant" much to the rousing delight of his collegiate audience, and while it is a time of the great political unrest in the United States due to the social reckoning of the civil rights movement and the antiwar protests, I am allowing myself to enjoy this idyllic and tranquil evening. The concert is part of my graduation celebration, and we are here to bask in the moment and to be immersed in the music.

Having graduated with mediocre grades and a degree in English Literature from a small Catholic college on the edge of New York City, which is primarily known for producing engineers and FBI agents—not writers and artists, I am filled with uncertainty about my future. I lack the funds and grades to pursue graduate training like most of my peers and, not having acquired any marketable skills for gainful employment, I am now a college graduate with no discernible plans or job offers. Admittedly, I'm feeling lost on this summer evening but, hey, at least, the music is good.

The emotional malaise I feel deepens over the next few months as I fruitlessly pursue leads through newspaper want ads and contacts provided by family and friends. Unfortunately, nothing has come of any of it, and I'm starting to feel discouraged that all of my schooling was for naught. But, as luck would have it, my dismal prospects seem to change the day I receive a notice in the mail from my college's career placement service. The government is about to administer the Federal Service Entrance Examination (FSEE), a test given to college graduates who are interested in employment with the federal government. With no other job prospects on the horizon, I sign up to take the exam. To my surprise, I score in the 99th percentile, which lands me a job as a management intern with a federal agency.

Six months into the training program, I find the unending clerical detail to be so intolerably mind numbing that I decide to resign. However, when I announce my intention to my training supervisor, Morgy, an impish balding man with wiry, black and gray hair who's been with the agency longer than anyone can remember, he asks me to delay my decision.

"Bob, there is a new special investigative unit being created within the agency," he says, pulling me into his office for privacy. "It's all very hush-hush but I think it might interest you, so, before you quit, I'd like you to meet with the man in charge of setting it up. His name is Charles Annibale."

Reluctantly, I delay my decision. Staying onboard for another week won't kill me, especially since no one is exactly banging down my door for me to come work for them. Later that week, I find myself sitting on a metal chair in an unfurnished suite of offices on the twenty-third floor of the federal building undergoing a lengthy interview. Opposite me is the person Morgy mentioned, Charles Annibale—a soft-spoken man in his late forties with short cropped prematurely white hair.

The interview lasts for several hours and consists of two parts. First, he scrutinizes my background and education, asking questions about my experience growing up in eastern Queens and my family relationships. He seems particularly interested that my father was a sergeant on the New York City police force for thirty years. The second part feels more like a test than an interview and involves me analyzing fact patterns in a series of scenarios and discussing their implications.

Finally, seeming to be satisfied with my responses, he leans forward on the metal desk, lacing his fingers together.

"Morgy was right about your analytical abilities. He always was a good talent spotter," he says, adjusting himself in his chair. "Bob, I'd like to offer you a job in the new unit that I am organizing for the agency to investigate fraud and corruption."

"Like doing law enforcement?" I ask naïvely.

"Well, not quite. We're not going after individuals. The agency already has other guys with guns and badges to do that. What we'll be doing is more like domestic intelligence work focused on organized corruption and fraud on federal contracts. This will be one of several investigative units of its type that are being set up across different agencies as we speak. There's one in Defense for military contracts and at Treasury for banks. The one I'm setting up will focus on civilian manufacturing and construction. You would be an agent in the field making observations, collecting data, and figuring out patterns so we can build a case. My impression is that you have the analytical skills to do the job, and I'll teach you the technical trade craft you'll need to survive on the street."

Agent in the field? Tradecraft? Survive on the street?

I nod like I know what he's talking about.

"What do you say?" he asks with his hand stretched across the table.

"Well, I'm tired of pushing papers around."

Charlie's eyes bore into me as he waits for my final answer.

"So, where do I sign up?" I ask with a toothy grin.

Charlie grabs my hand. "Good! Welcome aboard. Now let's go find some furniture for this place and get to work."

From that moment on, Charlie and I click. I later learn that he was a decorated World War II Navy vet who survived the sinking of his transport ship during the D-Day invasion. After the war, he graduated college and initially started working as an investigator for the Department of Defense. Later, he headed up investigative units for several federal agencies, some quite clandestine, before being asked to lead my agency's new investigative office.

Over the next eight years, Charlie does exactly what he promised in the interview. He initially teaches me the ins and outs of field work then expands into the craft of surveillance, investigative interviews, and how to cultivate and work with informants. Most importantly, though, he teaches me how to use statistics and records to analyze an organization's structure, activities, and finances. He is both my partner and mentor and occasionally acts as my protector within the agency, especially when my early twenties' idealism causes me to run afoul of its political and hierarchal power structure. Under his guidance, I learn to conduct investigations on the streets of New York and quickly discover that I have a knack for field work, especially data analysis.

As my status rises within the agency, I eventually become the unit's chief investigator, supervising a team of four other field agents. Hitting my stride, I confidently begin our next investigation into fraud concerning the construction of the addition to 26 Federal Plaza in lower Manhattan.

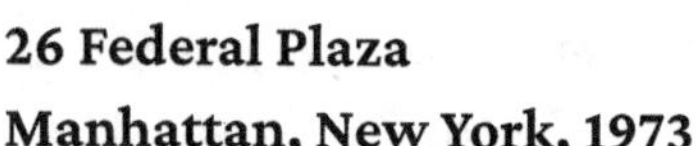

26 Federal Plaza
Manhattan, New York, 1973

It's Friday, and my team and I are sitting around the table in a small conference room. Amidst stacks of files, reports, and papers, we are wrapping up the details of a case involving a phony manufacturing company in the Bronx when, suddenly, Charlie bursts through the door.

"I just got a tip from one of my sources about no-show union jobs[8] here at 26 Federal Plaza," he says, breathing heavily. "The second phase of the building's addition is in full swing, and there's a lot of money involved and even more rumors about funds being diverted. I think this could be big. I want you and your team to drop everything else and start looking into this. I'll get you access to the site for surveillance and have accounting send you the financials."

Over the next three months, my team and I disguise ourselves as building inspectors to observe the day-to-day work on the construction site. I spend nights and weekends going over payroll records and time sheets. The walls of the conference room get covered with charts, diagrams, and lists. Finally, bleary-eyed on a late Friday afternoon surrounded by my team, I present our findings to Charlie.

"Your informant was right. The numbers just don't add up," I say. "The time sheets and payroll don't match the number of people we actually saw working on the construction site. We are paying for a lot of people who aren't there."

---

8. A "no show job" is a paid position for which no work, or even attendance, is actually expected. The awarding of no-show jobs is a form of political or corporate corruption.

My team nods in agreement.

"A lot!" I emphasize. "The scope of this fraud is staggering. It could amount to upwards of a million dollars on this project alone, and we haven't even looked at any of the other projects in the region where this might be going on. However, not every contractor on the project is involved. It all seems to involve just this one union."

Charlie spends the next week carefully examining our findings. By Friday morning, he calls me into his office, pointing to the pile of papers on his desk.

"I agree this is pretty damning stuff," he says grimly, "but I think before we present this to the U.S. Attorney, we should meet with the union's business agent to discuss our findings and see if he has a reasonable explanation for what we found."

"Seems like a good idea, Charlie. I'll set up the meeting for early next week before we go to Trenton to meet with the informant in that other manufacturing fraud case in Jersey."

He nods, and I leave his office to call the union's secretary to set up a meeting with the construction project's "business agent."

The following Tuesday, Charlie and I meet with the business agent in our conference room. The meeting starts off calmly as I present the findings to a squat man who is built like a heavyweight fighter with bulging neck muscles that spring from shoulders nearly touching his ears. He listens unmoved and disinterested.

"So? I don't see any problem," he responds gruffly. "You know, you shouldn't get involved in union business."

Perhaps it is the business agent's dismissive attitude or the subtle threat of his comment, but something in his response triggers Charlie. Without warning, he leaps from behind his desk and stands looming over the business agent. Leaning down, he points his finger in the man's face.

"Listen! Either this stops now, and the monies get paid back or we go to the U.S. Attorney and have him file an injunction barring your workers from the construction site until the matter is resolved."

The business agent's face suddenly turns blood red and two veins pop out of his thick neck muscles. He abruptly jumps toward Charlie. Fearing that there might be a physical altercation, I force myself between them. The business agent finally backs away after an uncomfortable stare down and storms out of the room.

"Yeah! We'll see about that!" he shouts.

Angry, Charlie picks up the phone and schedules a meeting with the Assistant U.S. Attorney. The meeting is set for the following Friday morning, since we'll be in Trenton on Thursday on another investigation. With our findings about to be handed off to the U.S. Attorney, I find myself happily thinking *Case closed.*

~

New Jersey Turnpike, 1973

As Charlie and I drive back to the city from Trenton after meeting with our informant, I glance over only to see that he's dosing off in the passenger seat of my 1970 mustard-yellow two-seater Triumph Spitfire convertible. With him sleeping, I'm left with my thoughts, the open road, and the radio to keep me awake. Turning my eyes back to the afternoon traffic in front of me, I stare blankly at the familiar stretch of the New Jersey Turnpike and fiddle with the radio dials trying to find a local FM station playing some rock or folk music to past the time. Eventually, my fingers find a college station playing Mike Oldfield's *Tubular Bells* when a massive jolt strikes the vehicle.

Disoriented, I feel like a gigantic fist hit me in the head and notice the car is rapidly accelerating. The speed pins my head against the bucket seat, and I instinctively press on the brakes, but the car continues to move. Unable to slow down, I look through the windshield as the highway begins to recede from underneath us. The steering wheel is moving in my hands, but the car doesn't respond. We're airborne.

With adrenaline kicking in, my stomach churns and bile rises in my throat. Time reverts to slow motion as our car veers off the side of the road. Out of my driver's side window, I see that we're careening into the ravine and brace myself for sudden death or, at the minimum, a life-altering injury. *This is going to hurt.*

The front of the car strikes the far side of the ravine first, and we become wedged between its walls. Thinking we've at least escaped death, I allow myself one deep breath before we begin to gator roll down the hill with bone-jarring thuds. *This is it.* With nothing but a soft convertible top to protect us, I prepare myself to be slammed into ground at the full force of gravity. *Thud!* I close my eyes. *Thud!* My knuckles turn white from squeezing the steering wheel. *Thud!*

Bracing for impact, I close my eyes as the car makes one final nosedive. *If there was ever a time to be wearing my seatbelt, this is it,* I think as the car eventually rolls itself (and us) right-side up.

Shaken and disoriented, I search for any sign of injury. After I scan my hands and body, I turn my attention to Charlie, whose upper body is now lying slumped over in my lap. *Oh God! He's dead.*

I reach my hand over to check for a pulse, but he lets out a low, anguished moan. I punch out both of our seat belts and pull him from the car, which now resembles a crumbled piece of yellow notepad paper.

Pulling Charlie to the edge of the road, he winces in pain. As I stroke his head trying to soothe him, I notice that traffic is ground to a halt on both sides of the turnpike. After several minutes, the flashing lights of a state police patrol car come toward us.

"What happened?" the trooper asks as the dizzying blur of the ravine rushing toward me flashes through my mind.

"I–We..." I mutter, unable to provide any coherent details except that my car suddenly accelerated and flew off the road. He looks on in disbelief.

I manage to say that we're federal investigators on our way back to Federal Plaza in New York City, but due to my irregular speech patterns, the state trooper crosses his arms and looks at me with narrowing eyes. That is, until a driver who witnessed the accident from the other side of the turnpike gives witness.

"I saw the whole thing. The little sports car was struck by a blue cargo van going about 100 miles per hour. It was like he was aiming for him. Struck him in the left rear and sent him flying. The van never stopped or decelerated. It just kept on going," the man says, his hands moving in short and sharp gestures.

Looking for evidence to support the witness's claim, the trooper walks down the highway and returns a few minutes later with the left rear taillight section of my convertible. It's covered in blue paint. I hold Charlie's hand as he looks up at me helplessly. The medics place him in an ambulance. His cold hands, pale face, and neck wrapped in a cervical collar sends a shiver down my spine.

Just before they lift him up, he grabs the coat of the trooper and asks the question on everyone's mind: "You don't think somebody did this on purpose, do you?"

The officer, who moments ago didn't believe us, remains silent, his gaze scanning the horizon.

~

26 Federal Plaza, 1973

I meet with Charlie to review the cause of the accident. He's still wearing the cervical collar and suffering from a post-concussive headache a week later.

Curious about what he said as they were putting him into the ambulance, I ask, "Charlie, why did you ask that state trooper if he thought somebody did this on purpose?"

He leans forward, placing both elbows on his desk. His face becomes cold, tense, and solemn.

"Because, Bob, it was an attempted hit. It turns out that the union is mobbed up. I've been on the phone all morning with the U.S. Attorney's Office. They are bringing in the FBI and launching a full investigation. They're convinced that what you found on the 26 Federal Plaza project is part of a much more widespread problem. They are going to meet with you later today to go over your findings on the building fraud and what you remember about our meeting with the business agent and the accident."

I panic. "My God, Charlie! A hit? That's crazy. Are you sure?"

"Pretty sure. They ran a background check on that business agent. He has a long record of arrests and has served time for assault and battery. He's basically a leg breaker[9] for the local mob. Bob, I grew up with these kinds of people on the lower East Side and have been dealing with them for a long time. They're dangerous, especially when money is involved, and we

---

9. Leg breaker: A violent thug, especially one employed as an enforcer by a criminal organization (e.g., a mafia or loan shark).

messed with their money—a lot of money as it turns out. And you don't mess with their money."

My mouth suddenly becomes dry with fear.

"Violence to them is just another tool in the toolbox like a drill or screwdriver," he continues, "and they use it with about as much feeling. Also, the timing makes sense to me since the accident happened before we had communicated our findings to the U.S. Attorney. If they had eliminated us, they would have eliminated our findings, too, and, *voilà*, no more problems," he says rubbing his palms together.

The pressure around my throat tightens like an anaconda's death grip. As if the emotional trauma from the accident weren't enough, knowing that this was an attempted hit creates a dread with me that I can't shake.

"You've got to be kidding!" I yell before covering my mouth and lapsing into a pensive silence.

Seeing that I'm quite shaken, Charlie stands up.

"You'll be doing interviews with the FBI for the rest of this week," he says, putting his arm around my shoulders. "But I've talked with our agency people in Washington, and we've agreed that you need to be out of the city until the FBI completes its investigation and indictments can come down. So, we're sending you on temporary assignment to the Puerto Rico field office until that happens. You'll probably have to come back to testify at some hearings, and I'll be in touch with you weekly. I want you to keep your head down while you're there. Understood?"

Sensing my dismay as I stare at the ground, he adds, "By the way, the U.S. Attorney said you did a great job with the investigation."

San Juan, Puerto Rico, 1974

Hiding in Puerto Rico for the six months it takes for the investigation to play out is not easy.

The FBI is able to determine that a blue cargo van entered the turnpike and took the nearest exit shortly after we went flying toward the ravine. However, neither the hitman nor the van was ever found, and the FBI agents speculate that since they were not successful in locating them, both the van and the driver are probably now buried somewhere in the wilderness of the New Jersey Pine Barrens[10].

This means that their investigation is unable to establish a connection between the accident and the business agent. They are, however, able to indict and convict him on multiple counts of contract fraud for the no-show schemes that he orchestrated on federal projects across the five boroughs of New York. He receives a long prison sentence, and the union local that he represented is temporarily placed under government receivership to reform its management and "business practices".

I keep a low profile in Puerto Rico doing surveillance and making only the essential trips to New York to testify, which leaves a lot of down time. I feel as though I've been exiled and especially miss the support of my fiancée, Astrid.

I have flashbacks of the accident along with violent images and vivid nightmares of Charlie and I plummeting to our death that jolt me awake in the middle of the night. I also develop an exaggerated startle reaction[11], especially when driving.

This is all exacerbated by paranoid thoughts of another

10. The Pine Barrens is a 1.1-million-acre National Reserve in southern New Jersey consisting mostly of vast undisturbed oak-pine forests (pine barrens) and wetlands.

11. Post-traumatic exaggerated startle response refers to an intense and heightened reaction to unexpected stimuli seen in individuals with post-trau-

attempted hit. I find myself wondering if the guy sitting next to me at the local bar or the woman at the next table in the restaurant is really on vacation having a drink or if they're here for a nefarious reason.

Trying to make sense of my feelings, I start re-reading Freud's *Outline of Psychoanalysis*. His theory on the inner workings of the human mind describes psychoanalysis as a technique that can bring about a cure to "the dreaded spontaneous illnesses of mental life"[12]. When I first read the book in a senior philosophy seminar, it had a profound impact on me and ignited my passion to become a psychotherapist, contrasting the otherwise dismal feelings of confusion and depression of my undergraduate years.

As I read the book again, it sings to me the same siren's song, proclaiming a truth I desperately need to hear: It's time to dust off the old college dream of becoming a psychotherapist. After college, I hesitated to pursue it because I felt that my poor grades and shallow academic background in psychology would eliminate me from the brutally competitive PhD admissions process. That, combined with my success as an investigator with Charlie, had relegated it to the backburner of my mind.

However, coming so close to death has shown me that my life can be snuffed out in an instant. The fact that I could have died on that highway has dramatically changed my perspective and made me realize that it's time to face my fears and pursue my dream, come what may. After many long phone calls with Astrid, who listens patiently as I work through my emotions, I come to the decision, which she whole heartedly

---

matic stress. It manifests as a sudden jump or flinch. It is indicative of an overactive stress response system and can be a persistent symptom.
12. Freud, S. (1949). P.24

supports, that I will pursue graduate training in clinical psychology and become a psychotherapist—a decision that will involve not only taking the prerequisite courses and exams but also leaving my secure position with the government and cashing in my pension along with everything I own to finance.

Federal Plaza, 1975

When I finally return to the New York office to resume my investigative duties, I feel an obligation to discuss this decision with Charlie. Sitting in the same chair when he shipped me off to Puerto Rico, I look at the man who's been a pivotal figure in my life since college, and a bittersweet sense of melancholy washes over me before I explain the revelations the accident has stirred within me.

Staring into the swirls of cream in my coffee, I open my mouth and sheepishly begin.

"Charlie, the accident and everything around it has caused me to take a deep look at what I want to do with my life. I love working with you, and you have taught me so much, but there is something I've wanted to do for a long time but have been too scared to try. I've decided to go to graduate school to become a psychologist and ultimately a psychotherapist."

Unexpectedly, Charlie sits back in his chair and smiles at me.

"Bob, I'm not surprised. You're a great investigator, and I've enjoyed our collaboration. I've also liked watching you grow since that day you came in as a young trainee. But I've known for a long time that you wanted to do something else. I don't think you know how much you have talked about it in our off moments together. So, no, I'm not surprised, and I'm glad you're finally going to do it. I am going to miss working with you and that crazy way you'd analyze the statistical patterns in our cases."

Taken aback that what I thought was just an internal struggle, I quickly interject.

"Well, it's not happening tomorrow. I'll be around for a while. I have a lot of things to do before I can get admitted to a program, but I just wanted you to know."

I stand up to shake his hand, but instead Charlie embraces me. Tears began welling up in both our eyes.

"Bob, you let me know if you need anything...anything," he says.

Over the next two years, while I continue working with Charlie, and even travel around the country training other investigators as part of a national taskforce for the agency, I complete the prerequisite courses and examinations and begin the complex and fiercely competitive admissions process for graduate school in clinical psychology.

Interestingly, when I'm finally accepted into the doctoral program at Long Island University (LIU), it turns out that my poor undergraduate grades didn't matter as much as I thought. It was the knowledge of statistical modeling and analysis I acquired as an investigator under Charlie's tutelage that aligns with the research interests of the graduate program's department chair. Turns out, he's in desperate need of a statistics teaching assistant and happily endorses my application—the very event that allows me to be standing behind this one-way mirror monitoring relapse rates among treated alcoholics.

THE GUILTY MECHANIC

> *"There is no human deed or thought that lies fully outside the experience of other people."*
>
> — IRVIN D. YALOM, 1995

MY CELTIC ANCESTORS engaged in an ancient ritual where a person, known as a sin-eater, would symbolically take on the sins of a deceased individual *allowing them to pass into the afterlife unburdened. As a psychotherapist, even though my approach to treating patients* is informed by my understanding of the neuroscience, to help them, I must be the holder of their darkest emotions and most horrible secrets, and in doing so, act much like these sin-eaters of old.

VA Medical Center

Newington, Connecticut, 1981

The young man sitting across from me in a generously padded office chair is slowly dying. His doctors are baffled by his condition. He has recurrent ulcers in his stomach and esophagus that are not responding to treatment, and he continues to bleed internally.

Outside of my office window, the oak trees that border the green meadow have begun to change into hues of amber and bright gold. It is fall in Connecticut, and the afternoon light is noticeably softer and no longer requires the blinds to be drawn as it did early in the summer when Billy[1] and I first began our therapy sessions.

It's been three and a half years since I left my position as a field agent with the agency. In the interim, I have completed the required academic training at LIU for my PhD in clinical psychology and am now doing my clinical internship treating patients at the Veteran's Administration Medical Center in Newington, Connecticut. I'm only in the fourth month of the 12-month psychotherapy program, and the seriousness of his condition scares me, but he is my patient, and I have to figure out a way to help him.

The patient before me is a man of average height in his mid-thirties with long unkempt brown hair and a full beard. Normally he dresses in jeans, a flannel shirt, and work boots for our sessions, but today he is in VA hospital pajamas, a robe, and slippers since he was admitted as an inpatient on the medical unit where the doctors are running tests on him. He is frightfully thin, and there are deep circles under his eyes, which give his face a haunted look and speak to the sleepless nights and nightmares he's had since coming to the hospital.

---

1. Name has been changed.

We've been working together since I began my internship, and it has taken every second of our time together for me to earn his trust.

Our initial treatment sessions were exceedingly difficult as he has been very taciturn, typically answering my questions with a shrug of the shoulders or one-to-two-worded answers. Many times, we simply sit in silence. While his VA records are filled with his medical history, they have not offered much background on him as a person. As a result, I do not yet have a good understanding of him psychologically or emotionally, except that he is profoundly sad, withdrawn, and angry.

Billy's war was Vietnam, a brutal jungle guerrilla war, which while fought abroad, had karmic effects that were felt in the United States' own backyard. Amidst the social upheaval at home, the soldiers who fought were treated quite poorly when they returned from their service. By the time Billy and I meet, these veterans have not only found their voice but are also pouring into the VA system in need of services.

As a group, they are quite distinct from the World War II and Korean veterans, which the VA is accustomed to treating. For one, Vietnam veterans are a lot more hostile because of how they are treated by the public who often referred to them as "baby killers" when they returned. There are also horror stories floating around in the media about the poor and deteriorated conditions of the VA facilities, especially the larger ones, where they have to come for treatment.

Complicating matters further, many of the veterans are exhibiting symptoms of post-traumatic stress disorder (PTSD). This is a relatively new psychiatric diagnosis, and our understanding of its complexities and treatment are still in their infancy.

Thankfully for Billy and I, the Newington VA Medical Center is quite small by VA standards. Located in a quaint New

England town just outside of Hartford, Connecticut, its red brick colonial building complete with a white dome and a bell tower is surrounded by an idyllic setting of green lawns and old oak and coniferous trees. It seems like an inviting and friendly place to my jaded New York eyes. The staff also treats their patients, including the Vietnam veterans, like family no matter how difficult their afflictions. Like most VA Medical Centers, it's also associated with major medical research at universities—in this case the University of Connecticut Medical School at West Hartford.

Despite Billy's guardedness during this initial phase of his treatment, I've been able to piece together a vague outline of his history both before his military service and during his deployment in Vietnam.

He grew up in a small New England town halfway between Hartford and the Massachusetts's border, a place of traditional values far from the 1960s cultural revolution and the war protests. His father owned the local auto repair shop in town, and Billy was trained in the family business of fixing vehicles. He and his father enjoyed building and racing stock cars together.

As an Eagle Scout, he was also a proud patriot of his country. His father served in the Army in Korea and his grandfather in World War II, so when the Vietnam war started heating up, he enlisted. For him, just as he had fixed cars, he felt going into the military was a family tradition and recalled that his father was proud of his decision.

Because of his mechanical aptitude and experience fixing cars, he was assigned to the motor pool and rose quickly through the ranks after basic training. He soon became a sergeant, and when he was finally deployed to Vietnam, he was assigned to run the motor pool unit at a forward ops base in a remote section of the country.

However, when I try to explore his experience in Vietnam, he stubbornly refuses to discuss it. Any attempt to explore his past is met with an uneasy and uncomfortable silence and usually results in the session ending early.

Over the years, patients have often shared horrible secrets with me. This usually occurs when they feel safe enough to open up, but the timing varies widely from person to person. For some, the process takes a few weeks and, for others, months or even years. Conversely, some patients divulge their deepest feelings in the first session as an immediate release, but then never return or commit to the therapeutic process. Being able to predict when any of this will occur has always eluded me, but I am certain that it's the repeated conversations over time that lead to a semblance of normalcy and recovery for most patients.

The process of psychotherapy is not as dramatic as it's portrayed in movies. While there are tense moments, the session-to-session conversations can involve topics as inconsequential as the weather, politics, or even sports. To some, this may seem irrelevant, but nothing in my experience that occurs in therapy is ever insignificant. Everything that happens in a treatment session highlights something new about the patient even though, at times, it may not be clear how each dot is connected. For me, the therapeutic process is cumulative with each new bit of data adding clarity to the patient's mosaic.

As Billy enters my office today, his countenance is noticeably different than in prior sessions. His guardedness, usually so prominent, has been replaced by a tense nervousness, which is physically palpable.

"Hi, Billy. How are you feeling?" I ask as he sits down.

Normally Billy responds with "fine" and then retreats into silence until I prompt him with another question or comment. Today, though, he doesn't give his routine response but simply stares out the window of my office. The physical tension emanating from his body does not suggest detachment from reality to me but rather an inner turmoil—a sense that he's coming to a difficult decision.

After what feels like an eternity, he looks at me and makes eye contact, which has been rare over the last few months. In this moment of prescient silence, I recognize that the time for sharing his secret has come. He is now ready—desperate even—to talk.

In a soft, nearly inaudible voice, he begins.

"You know, fall in Vietnam is not like it is here. It is very different," he says before pausing.

In every therapy session, there are inflection points. These are moments that mark a transition in the working relationship between patient and therapist. What often starts as an awkward and anxious greeting turns into a handshake when both parties decide to work together. This sometimes evolves into the occasional moment when both individuals are both brought to tears out of profound sadness or raucous laughter at something absurd.

One of the most significant inflection points is when the patient begins to trust their therapist enough to reveal their deepest and most private secrets. The office décor and past conversations all fade into the background as the patient finally faces their demons. Such moments leave me emotionally drained and in a deeply reflective state not only about their personal experiences but also about my own.

The next 90 minutes unfold seamlessly as Billy shares the extraordinary story of his experience in Vietnam. It's a powerful moment, but, more importantly, it begins to give me the keys to understanding what's happening to him physically.

"It was late 1968, just after Tet[2]," he continues, his voice now louder and clearer. "Everybody was on high alert and a bit paranoid. We saw North Vietnamese and Viet Cong behind every tree and in every shadow. I was stationed at this forward ops base, which had already been attacked once. Lots of secret stuff and special ops going on that I didn't know much about. I was in charge of the motor pool. My job was to keep the trucks running, so we could supply the units that were really far out in the boonies. I was good at it and had a great team of guys. We were all really close. I guess like part of a family or a brotherhood. Then, it all went to hell."

Billy pauses as he relives the most traumatic moment of his life. His breathing becomes rapid. His hands are clenched into fists. His jaw tightens. Then, trying to suppress his emotions, he closes his eyes and takes a deep breath. I can sense his anguish and know that we are about to get into something dark and terrible.

"They all got killed," he whispers, looking into his lap.

I take a deep breath to absorb the shock.

"It had been relatively quiet for several weeks. Not even the occasional mortar round. So, the orders came down to resupply some of the more remote forward outpost camps. I prepared two trucks, and a jeep escort mounted with an M60 machine gun. Two men to each truck and three in the jeep. All armed. They set out in the pre-dawn. We had expected them back by the early afternoon, but time came and went with no

---

2. Tet - The Tet Offensive was a surprise attack on 30 January 1968 by The Viet Cong and North Vietnamese People's Army of Vietnam, against the forces of the South Vietnamese, The United States and their allies launched. It was major escalation and one of the largest military campaigns of the Vietnam War.

contact. I knew that things happened in the field. Trucks could break down or get damaged, which could delay things. They had walkie-talkies, but these were notoriously unreliable. Still, as time went on with no communication, I became more and more worried."

He pauses for a few seconds, rubbing his hands against his legs.

"It was near dusk when a lone soldier from the jeep escort stumbled back into camp. He was wounded and bleeding but still had managed to walk almost 10 klicks[3] back. He said they had been ambushed halfway to the outpost. He thought some type of IED[4] had taken out the forward truck but wasn't sure because it all happened so fast. He said there were all these explosions and then they were being shot at from everywhere. Both sides of the road and in front and in back of them. He then got knocked out by an explosion, and when he woke up, he said everything was silent and the enemy was gone. In a daze, he had just started walking back to camp. Then, sobbing, he said, 'Everybody is dead.'"

Billy stares into space as his eyes turn glassy.

"What happened next?" I ask.

He looks down at the floor, resting his elbows on his knees.

"The next morning, we sent out a heavily armed patrol with two armored vehicles to assess the scene and recover the bodies of our buddies. They came back with the casualties but did not encounter either the North Vietnamese or Viet Cong. They reported that there were clear signs of an intense fire fight but did not see any evidence of the enemy being wounded. Both trucks and the jeep had been totally disabled."

---

3. "Klicks" - In the military, one klick equals one kilometer, which is approximately 0.62 miles.

4. IED: improvised explosive device

At this point I can sense the same of inner turmoil welling up in him as when he began the session. He fights through his emotions, trying to suppress his anger as he clenches his teeth and begins to rock back and forth.

"My 22-year-old newly commissioned lieutenant told me to send out two flatbed tow trucks to haul in the damaged trucks and to tow the jeep behind. He didn't think an armed escort would be necessary since the armored patrol hadn't seen any signs of the enemy. I argued with him. I had just lost six of my men! But he overruled me, saying that those were his orders, and I was to follow them. The next morning, I sent out two flatbeds each with a crew of three but no armed jeep escort. Given the kind of damage that had been described, I figured half a day to get the equipment back."

Billy's voice breaks as his tone shifts from anger to anguish.

"It was dusk when we got the call this time. It had been a trap with the trucks as bait. There was another intense fire fight going on and my men were trapped. We sent out a rapid response team with an armored vehicle, but it was too late. Five of my six men were dead, but the sixth was oddly...no, miraculously...unharmed. Badly shaken but not a scratch."

Billy's hands are tightly clenched, and his face looks like a contorted Freddy Krueger Halloween mask from the physical tension he's experiencing.

"In 72 hours, I had lost 11 men. That was almost half my unit. I was so angry. I wanted to kill the people who did this. I wanted to find them and kill them in the most gruesome way I could think of," he says, slamming his fists against his leg.

As I listen and observe his body language, I find myself swept away in his emotions. My heart begins to race, and I am suddenly overwhelmed with the same sense of profound sadness and grief, or, in this case, the intense rage that envelops Billy. This is an experience that occasionally happens in treatment. Unlike the dictionary definition of empathy, which is simply to understand or relate to the feelings of another person, this is different. I am directly experiencing Billy's emotional pain.

Continuing, Billy says, "It was then that my lieutenant did something that was incomprehensible to me. He brought the soldier who had survived up on charges. Something about cowardice and dereliction of duty. He was blaming him for the mess that *he* had created. When I heard this, I snapped and got a grenade. I was going to frag[5] him in his tent that night. I was so full of rage. It was so wrong what he was doing, but my guys stopped me from killing him. They got me drunk, and I fell asleep. When I woke up the next morning, the rage was gone, but I felt very strange. Detached. No emotion. Nothing. Everything seemed familiar but also felt surreal at the same time."

At this, Billy pauses, and an eerie feeling comes over me. I can't quite put my finger on it. I can sense that his mood has dramatically shifted, but when he starts speaking again, it sounds as if his words are coming from someone else. The sadness and grief that consumed him a few moments ago are gone. In its place, another emotion is building.

As the tension rises in the room, it's clear that he is being overtaken by these new emotions, and they aren't just about the war, the ambush of his friends, or even the actions of his lieutenant. They are about something else, something more sinister.

"I don't recall having a plan the next day, but I requisitioned a jeep and drove out of the base beyond the last of the fences and tripwires that were supposed to keep us safe. I think

---

5. Frag: *Fragging* is the deliberate or attempted killing of a soldier, usually a superior officer, by a fellow soldier. U.S. military personnel coined the word during the Vietnam War, when such killings were most often committed or attempted with a fragmentation grenade.

I had some idea of going to the scene of the ambush. It seemed to me that I drove for a long time until I came upon the killing field. On the side of the road was the burned-out wreckage of trucks, jeeps, and flatbeds. I got out of my jeep and wandered around. All around me I could see the blood spatter where my men had been killed," he says, sobbing. "It was horrible. They were my guys. I had lived with them, trained them, ate with them, drank with them, shared stories about our lives and families back home. And now they were just red brown smudges in the clay and grass."

His voice is now distorted as his emotions begin to break through.

"Billy, take a deep breath, hold it, and slowly let it out," I instruct.

Unfortunately, this is like suggesting that a runaway loco-motive slow down. I, too, feel myself caught up in the emotions that are erupting in him. I feel them as deeply as if I were there with him on the jungle road. His murderous rage swells within me, and the intensity of it stuns and frightens me.

"I don't know how long I stayed there looking at the scene, but I eventually got back in my jeep and began driving again. As I drove, the jungle gave way to open farmland and rice paddies. I recall the sunlight reflecting off the water in them. I don't remember hearing any sounds. The sunlight and the quiet all felt surreal because my head was on fire with images of blood and wreckage and a terrible desire to find the people who did this and kill them."

The hackles on the back of my neck go up. My intuition is screaming. *Something dreadful is coming. Be alert!*

"After a time, I came upon a field in which two peasants were working in one of the paddies. They saw me and one of them waved. I think to signal that they were "friendlies", not

Viet Cong. I don't know for sure. I can't recall thinking anything really. I was just feeling this intense anger. Then everything becomes very dreamlike, and I see myself from afar getting out of my jeep and taking my rifle walking to the edge of the road and shooting them both. It was like watching a movie. I can see me doing it, but it doesn't seem like me somehow."

Tears are now flowing down his face, and his voice has become distorted as his rage is replaced by a choked anguished wail.

"I killed those two men. They weren't doing anything. They weren't the enemy. They were just planting rice, and I killed them. I can see them now, as I have seen them every day since then."

Billy stops talking as he slumps forward in the chair, face in hands, weeping. I sit in a dazed silence while my mind races. The emotional tsunami of what I've just heard washes over me. *My patient just told me that he murdered two people in cold blood.*

At this point, it is me who is taking and slowly letting out deep breaths. I can feel the pain that Billy is experiencing becoming a part of me and I'm viscerally affected by his words just as if I were standing there with him on the edge of the jungle staring at the horror of those two dead farmers.

His actions are at the core of what's been emotionally and physically torturing him for over a decade. However, I am his psychotherapist, not his judge. It is my role to help him navigate his trauma, and determinations about the morality or legality of his actions are for someone else in another space and time.

As his emotions settle, Billy's tone turns dry.

"Afterward, I got back in my jeep and drove back to the base. I didn't tell anyone what I'd just done. There was never any report about finding the bodies of farmers from anyone else. I guess you could chalk it up to the "fog of war" and all that. Until now, it has been my secret. You are the only person I've ever told."

I allow him to have the last word, and there is a deafening silence in the room as I continue to struggle to absorb what he has just told me. In the silence, the axiom of the great psychiatrist Harry Stacks Sullivan becomes my guiding mantra.

"We are all much more simply human than otherwise, be we happy and successful, contented and detached, miserable and mentally disordered, or whatever."

With this thought comes the realization that at the core of Billy's pain is not just the result of his actions that day but the loss of his *shared humanity.* No matter what treatment strategies I develop to address his symptoms, I have to manage this issue if I'm going to truly help him. I recognize that this will require me to join him on his journey, but when the session ends, I feel drained and troubled. Even so, as the holder of his darkest secret, it's still up to me to figure out how to help him.

In becoming a psychotherapist, clinical supervision is one of the most important parts of the training process. Clinical supervisors teach the novice therapist the subtleties and nuances of working with patients. The first clinical supervisor often plays a foundational role not only in how the young therapist comes to understand and deliver treatment but also in the overall trajectory of their career. Fortunately for me, that individual is Dr. Eugene B. Daniels.

Billy's disturbing revelations and my own uncertainty about how to treat him are the subject of my next supervision session with Dr. Daniels. Like most young psychotherapists, I naïvely search for some clever intervention that will "fix" Billy.

However, Dr. Daniels tends to be more Socratic[6] in his approach, raising questions for me to explore rather than simply giving me concrete or fixed responses. He also has two characteristics that I have tried to emulate: empathy for the emotional experience supervisee and objectivity when observing the clinical conditions and symptoms the patient presents.

He begins this supervision session by helping me explore my emotional reaction to Billy's revelation.

"A very strange and disturbing story, Bob. How did it make you feel?"

"I guess I was shocked initially. You know, Dan, I saw a lot of screwed up things when I was on the street with the feds. People doing all sorts of dirty deals for money. Hell, I almost got killed over it. So, I've dealt with people who are seriously violent, but I never talked to anyone who actually told me they murdered someone. That's why I think what Billy told me shocked me at first."

"And was there anything else you felt, Bob?"

"Well, sadness," I reply, surprised by the simplicity of his question. Dan pauses, allowing me to come to a sobering realization about my own anger.

"That war! Such a waste and for what?" I suddenly shout. "Just lots of dead bodies and ruined lives on all sides. I lost a number of close friends. They just went off to war and never came back and the ones who did were changed by it. Even my best childhood friend, Mayo. We grew up together in the same small town in Queens. Went to the same Catholic elementary

---

6. Socratic: The Socratic Method is a dialogue-based learning technique that stimulates critical thinking and self-discovery through questioning.

and high school. We ran track together and romanced the same girls. We were like brothers."

Suddenly, I'm invaded by memories of Mayo, the war, and the emotions I'd long forgotten—*or repressed?*

Like Billy, Mayo enlisted in the military out of a sense of duty. He was a paratrooper with the famed 503rd Airborne Infantry Regiment and had been wounded as a forward observer[7] in a fire fight.

When he returned, I went to visit him. We were sitting in the same bedroom in his house that we had in high school listening to Bob Dylan and Joan Baez fantasying about our futures, but he was no longer the funny, adventurous, and optimistic guy I knew from childhood. He was bitter, angry, and withdrawn.

As we sat there in his room, I could see his full dress uniform with its corporal stripes, a chest full of ribbons and a purple heart hanging in a clear plastic bag on his closet door. However, when I told him that I was impressed by all his accolades and medallions, his face grew grim, and he responded to my observation with a frightening coldness in his voice that I had never heard in all our years as friends.

"I hate it. I hate what it represents. I hate what I did over there and how it has changed me," he said just moments before his voice fell silent.

After that day, we never sat in that bedroom again. While I would occasionally visit him over the next few years, our friendship was never the same. My childhood friend had never returned from the war.

------

7. Forward Observer: A soldier who goes into hostile territory or a forward position on the battlefield to identifying targets, direct artillery and mortar fire and gather intelligence for use in operations. Considered one of the most dangerous jobs in the military, *forward observers* are subjected to a rigorous selection and training process.

The revelation that Billy's emotions were a reflection of my own suppressed rage felt like taking a punch to the gut.

"So, you felt anger as you listened to Billy talk!" Dr. Daniels exclaims. "Anger about what happened to Billy and to your friend Mayo. Normal kids who were caught up in that unimaginable horror. What else do you think Billy was feeling as he told you, his secret?"

"Oh! He was angry too!" I say with an unyielding resoluteness. "But there was also intense guilt and pain. So much pain. He couldn't undo what happened to his men or what he did to those farmers, and he couldn't tell anyone. He's had to hold it inside, and it became like a poison that's slowly killing him!"

"So, you see your patient is in pain and feeling helplessness. What did that make you feel?"

"I felt his pain and rage! It was like it was *in* me. It was so intense. I just wanted it to stop. Then, I thought to myself, *He is my patient, and I am supposed to make it stop for him,* but I didn't know how to make it stop. I felt so helpless."

"Exactly, you felt the pain, rage, and helplessness that he was feeling. It was not just about what you heard but what you felt. It is natural for us as humans to avoid such feelings, however, as a psychotherapist, it is important not only to be both aware of what the patient is feeling but also what their feelings make you feel and then to use it as a tool in the treatment process. It provides you with almost direct knowledge of your patient's inner experience. Based on what you have just told me about Billy, I believe it is essential for you to continue to experience and understand what he's going through if you are going to help him change the way he deals with his emotions."

Dr. Daniels shifts in his chair as if something is making him physically uncomfortable. His chest rises and falls as he rapidly inhales. Then he slowly exhales before speaking again. There's a subtle change in his voice. His professorial tone is gone, replaced by one that feels more personal—almost sad and weary.

"It is also the hardest and most exhausting part of our job. It is not easy to allow yourself to feel what someone else is feeling. You pay an emotional and a physical price."

Leaning forward and placing both his hands on the arm rest of his leather chair, he stares directly into my eyes.

"But it is one of the most powerful experiences you will ever have with your patient in psychotherapy."

Having stressed the importance of developing a nuanced understanding of my and Billy's emotional landscape, he retreats, shifting the focus of our conversation to Billy's post-traumatic stress and physical symptoms.

"The post-traumatic stress disorders that these Vietnam vets are presenting with are new to all of us. They don't fit our traditional clinical models, and we are still figuring out how to treat them. Vietnam was a different type of war than World War II and Korea. It was a jungle guerilla war, and their responses to this have been different. However, the physical symptoms that Billy is having and their severity are highly unusual, even for these vets. There is clearly trauma here, but what is going on with him is more complex and puzzling. It sounds like there is also a somatic[8] conversion of some type involved in which all that grief, emotional pain, and guilt have somehow been converted into physical symptoms."

Searching for the quick fix, I ask, "So, what's the strategy to treat post-traumatic stress with a somatic conversion?"

"Bob, psychotherapy is a very intimate individualized process between the therapist and the patient," he replies, not taking the bait. "What's going on with Billy is very complex

---

8. Somatic: Relating to the body as opposed to the mind.

and there is no canned or cookie cutter[9] approach that's going to work. You are going to have to figure it out with him. However, I can tell you that among my colleagues here, there is considerable interest in the long-term physical effects of stress and its role in creating psychopathology. You might want to look at the clinical literature on stress to figure out what is going on with Billy in order to develop specific therapeutic strategies to treat him."

I nod in agreement.

"As your clinical supervisor, however, what I do know is that he trusted you enough to share his story, his secret, and, in my experience, that trust is always part of the cure no matter the specific problem or treatment. So, keep listening and helping him to share his feelings, even if it is hard for you to hear it sometimes."

While Dr. Daniels hasn't given me the quick fix that I wanted, his advice about reviewing the clinical literature on stress activates the investigator in me with a new insight. *To help Billy, I have to solve the puzzle between the stress caused by his war-time experiences and his physical symptoms. This will require not just talking with him but also doing research like I used to do for the government, putting the pieces together into an understandable pattern.*

Energized by these thoughts, I drive, perhaps, a little too fast, to the medical school's library and begin researching stress and its effects on neurological, psychological, and physical functioning. Huddled over a small desk surrounded by a pile of books and research papers, I study the work of Hungarian endocrinologist, Hans Selye.

---

9. A canned cookie cutter approach refers to a standardized method or solution that is applied uniformly across different situations without consideration of unique needs or contexts.

Selye, who originally coined the term "stress" in 1936, became fascinated with this issue early in his medical career after observing physical responses in seriously ill patients that were not the direct result of their disease but related to the generalized stress their illnesses caused. He later became famous for a series of experiments in which he exposed laboratory animals to chronic stress and found significant changes to their internal organs. The changes he observed included damage to the adrenal glands, atrophy of the lymphatic system including the thymus, and, of most interest to me because of Billy's physical symptoms, the development of peptic ulcers in the stomach and duodenum.

Selye's belief was that in addition to any specific action taken in coping with a situational threat, the body has a nonspecific, generalized "stress response." He went on to describe this response as a "general adaptation syndrome," more commonly referred to as "Selye's Syndrome." It involved a three-part process: an *alarm phase* (also called a fight-or-flight reaction), a *resistance phase* (in which the body tries to recover) and, if the stressor continues, an *exhaustion phase*.

He found that in the *alarm phase*, people experienced a hormonal release, particularly from the adrenal glands, that caused specific physical symptoms, including increases in heart, respiration rates, and blood pressure. In the *resistance phase*, the body tried to repair itself after the initial shock of stress. If the stressful situation was no longer present, their heart, respiration rates, and blood pressure would start to return to prestress levels. However, if the stress continued, the body never returned to normal "prestress" functioning levels and continued to secrete stress hormones. Since chronic exposure to stress hormones is harmful to the body, this leads to the *exhaustion phase* where the body's physical, emotional, and mental resources are depleted and physical organ damage begins.

I find his description of this syndrome and particularly, the characteristics of the *exhaustion phase,* to be useful in understanding what's going on with Billy. However, Selye's findings were primarily describing the direct effects of prolonged physical stress, not the delayed effects of psychological stress. Also, because he was mostly dealing with animal subjects and didn't account for the emotional and cognitive centers of the human brain, I find this area to be one I need to explore with regards to Billy's somatic symptoms. While Selye's work gives me general understanding of what Billy's experiencing, it does not identify the specific trigger for his stress that I can help him manage.

Billy sits opposite from me in the late afternoon sunlight. As he elaborates on the aftermath of the murder of the two farmers, his body posture and facial expression lack the tension and stiffness they previously had. He even seems eager to talk and picks up the discussion from where he left without any prompting.

"After I shot them, I recall feeling emotionally numb for several weeks. I just kept everything inside. I couldn't tell anybody about what I'd done. Then I started having episodes during the day when I would relive everything, like I was watching myself in a movie. I also began having these nightmares where I would wake up in a cold sweat in the middle of the night consumed with feelings of guilt and shame."

Curious, I ask, "Didn't anybody notice the change in you?"

"No. No one seemed to notice. Even when I wasn't much good at doin' my motor pool job anymore, they didn't notice. I eventually rotated home a few months later and got an honorable discharge for duty in time of war."

"What was it like after you got home?"

"After I got home, I couldn't pick up the pieces. Couldn't talk about the war and definitely not about what I had done although I think my family could see the change in me. Kept to myself mostly. I tried drinking but it made things really bad, so I don't drink anymore. Couldn't work with my dad either. Working on cars just brought back the memories and the flashbacks. A few years later, I started getting sick with the ulcers and bleeding inside. It's been a long time since I've felt well."

"Billy, when you relive the memories now, what's that like?"

"When the memories come back, I can't make sense of them. It's like I was one person before everything happened and another afterward. I know I really wanted to kill that lieutenant, but I didn't, and I didn't have any reason to kill those farmers, but I did. I still relive it every day and every night, and when I do, I know it's me, but it oddly feels like it's *not* me."

What strikes me is Billy's use of the phrase "not me." Because he couldn't share what happened with anyone, he's bottled up the secret, creating an intense emotional energy that's caused a split of his identity—the Billy before the murder and the Billy after.

Billy has internalized the guilt and trauma, and these emotions are what's triggering his flashbacks and nightmares. What he *externalized* are the memories, especially the one of him murdering the two innocent farmers. This moment feels alien to him because his brain cannot integrate his actions into his sense of self, making him unable to process what occurred emotionally. This has resulted in an unresolvable stress and, like Selye postulated, an overproducing of the stress hormones, which is causing his psychological and physical illness.

With these thoughts in mind, I am beginning to understand the nature of his emotional conflict and his physical illness.

In my clinical experience, the phrase "not me" is often used by patients who engage in uncharacteristic behaviors during a traumatic event. Because their actions are emotionally devasting for them, their minds create a separation from reality, also known as disassociation, to such an extent that their actions feel carried out by someone else entirely. These acts can include engaging in impulsive sex, drug use, or harrowing acts of rage and violence as with Billy.

The psychiatrist Sullivan discusses the evolution of the *not me* in his developmental theory. He posits that because of the infant's existential dependency on others for their survival, the child quickly develops a sense of behaviors and experiences that are associated with a "good" and a "bad" version of themselves. The integration over time of these associations into the child's identity eventually creates their sense of "right and wrong," otherwise known as their conscience. However, he also postulated that this same existential dependency creates another range of behaviors and emotions that the child labels as *not me*. These are behaviors that are so disruptive to their dependency relationships that they pose a threat to individual's survival.

He believed that the emotional driver for the development of *good me, bad me*, and *not me* was the anxiety level of the infant. *Good me* is associated with a state of little to no anxiety whereas *bad me* contains mild to moderately severe anxiety. However, the *not me* behaviors are associated with an extreme, catastrophic form of anxiety called annihilation anxiety[10] in which the child feels that their very existence is threatened.

From a neuropsychological perspective, there is strong evidence to support this theory of human development. While the human brain's neuroanatomic structure is incredibly complex, from an evolutionary perspective it can be divided into two parts: the neocortex, or the "new" brain (sometimes thought of as the "thinking brain") and the paleomammalian cortex, the "old" brain (sometimes referred to as the "rat brain").

The terms "new" and "old" in this classification refer to the order in which the two different parts of the brain evolved over time. The paleomammalian cortex, which plays a critical role in ensuring the survival of the organism and the procreation of its species, developed first. The neocortex developed later to regulate the paleomammalian cortex and is associated with language production, complex information processing, logical reasoning, and emotional regulation. Anatomically, the paleo-mammalian cortex is located in the core part of the brain with the much larger neocortex sitting both above and around it just under the top of the skull.

In the service of survival and procreation, the paleomam-malian cortex manages the numerous biological processes occurring in the body such as cardiovascular function, temper-ature regulation, digestion, respiration, and hormonal func-tioning. More importantly, it also controls our fight, flight, and freeze responses by generating emotions such as fear and anxiety to alert the neocortex so that humans take the neces-sary steps to survive any threat.

The survival benefit of these paleomammalian emotional

---

10. *Annihilation anxiety* is a deep-seated fear of losing one's sense of self or ceasing to exist, often triggered by trauma or overwhelming stress.

inputs is that the neocortex develops neural networks that detects behaviors that help us meet our basic needs and avoid potentially unpleasant and dangerous situations before they occur. This is similar to having a list of "do's" (Sullivan's *good me*) and "don'ts" (his *bad me*) that help humans avoid pain, suffering, and severely traumatic experiences including death. Over time, the *good me* and *bad me* become integrated into one's sense of self, and humans learn to avoid situations or actions that activate the *bad me* versions of themselves. They are also drawn toward people and situations that align with the *good me* identity. In Billy's case, enlisting in the army was the *good me* version of himself. However, his actions in murdering the two farmers are associated with an unbearable anxiety, which threatens his existence simply because he cannot integrate them into his sense of self.

Even though it is both dwarfed in size and processing capacity by the neocortex, the paleomammalian cortex has the capacity to take over one's entire neurological system under certain situations. Referred to as limbic hijacking[11], this process occurs in situations that typically involve a threat to the survival of the individual or those close to them—situations including disasters, accidents, assaults, abuse, serious medical events, and, in Billy's case, war.

In these situations, the primitive brain briefly takes control of the neocortex and the nervous system. The individual will then engage in automaton-like behavior that involves a high degree of dissociation or loss of awareness[12] of their behaviors

---

11. Limbic or emotional hijacking refers to a rapid and overwhelming emotional reaction that bypasses rational thinking and can lead to impulsive behavior or irrational decisions. During an emotional hijacking the part of the brain responsible for emotional processing takes control and overrides the neocortex, which is responsible for logical reasoning and decision-making.

12. Dissociation is a disruption in how the mind processes information that

and emotions. Patients I've worked with describe events like these as similar to having an "out-of-body experience" in which the situation takes on a dreamlike quality, and they observe their actions as if they were being performed by an impostor.

Unfortunately, though, there is no impostor and, if an individual in response to limbic hijacking engages in *not me* behaviors, there are significant repercussions beyond dissociation. Since these behaviors, as Sullivan posits, are associated with unbearable anxieties and cannot be integrated into their sense of self, they cause an unresolvable emotional conflict that triggers the *Selye syndrome.*

For me, this explains the origin of Billy's somatic symptoms. Having engaged in *not me* behaviors during an episode of limbic jacking, he's subjected to a chronic state of intense and unbearable anxiety and partially dissociates from it. However, while understanding this is helpful, it does not provide me with a therapeutic strategy to help him resolve his conflict. I will need to explore and change how he processes emotional information and triggers—something he's already given me clues on how to do.

One of my mentors during graduate training at Long Island University, Dr. John Exner, believed that humans could be divided into three groups. For him, individuals who externalize their emotional responses were *Extratensives*; those who internalized them were *Introversives,* and those who vacillated

---

causes an individual to feel disconnected from their thoughts, feelings, memories, and surroundings. It can be triggered by stress or trauma as well as biological or biochemical factors.

between internalization and externalization were *Ambitents*. He felt that each processing style had its advantages in handling difficult situations but that each also contained liabilities that could lead to the development of psychological and emotional problems. For example, *Extratensives* tend to be more vulnerable to impulsive behaviors while *Introversives* can have trouble identifying their emotions. They're also at a higher risk for depression and experiencing physical symptoms associated with stress. While these processing mechanisms typically become fixed in the individual by adulthood, he believed that they could be modified with treatment.

While Billy would be classified as an *Introversive* in this system, his difficulty in perceiving and describing his emotions suggests the presence of a clinical condition called *Alexithymia* (Latin for *without words for emotions*)[13]. His *Introversive* style set the stage that day in the killing fields of Vietnam. The combination of the *not me* behaviors and the involuntary suppression of his emotions prevented him from processing the trauma. This led to chronic and acute stress symptoms, ultimately leading to Selye's *exhaustion phase* and the development of his ulcers.

With these insights, I feel my clinical analysis of Billy's problem is complete, and I can now craft his treatment plan. The confession itself was therapeutic for Billy, and it's the first real step in his treatment. Now, though, I have to work with him on recognizing and expressing his emotions. As he becomes more skilled, we can then begin to integrate his dissociated emotions from the trauma and hopefully reduce the chronic stress that's causing his ulcers.

---

13. Alexithymia is a personality trait that makes it hard to feel, understand, and express emotions.

Billy is more willing to engage in conversation after divulging his secret. In some ways, he even seems chatty. However, he still has significant difficulty in recognizing and expressing his emotions—so much so that our conversations often feel superficial.

I initially focus on having him recognize his emotions since he does not do so naturally. This requires me to observe his movements, body posture, and micro-expressions and ask him questions about what he's feeling.

During the next treatment session, Billy describes his relationship with his father after he returned from Vietnam and begins to look off into space with his eyes downcast.

"Billy, what are you feeling right now?" I ask.

"Oh! I was remembering how my dad and I worked on cars together."

Pointing first to my head, I say, "No, that's what you were thinking, Billy. What does it feel like in here?" I ask, tapping the middle of my chest.

"I miss him. He died a few years ago, and I never was able to work with him like before. I was feeling sad."

"Yes, you were feeling sad," I say, reinforcing the connection between his emotion and its name.

After we have repeated this process a number of times, I start training him on describing his feelings outside of treatment starting with minor interactions between him and people from his small town. Billy first recognizes the feeling of frustration when the local drug store gives him the wrong medications. On another day, he describes feeling joy when he saw the foliage changing on the trees in front of his family's home.

As he becomes more proficient in identifying his own

emotions, I have him identify what he perceives to be other people's emotions. In one instance, I asked him what he felt when he saw a mother scolding her crying child in a grocery store to which he eagerly replied, "I knew what that child felt! He was sad and frightened!"

These exercises teach him a new language. Much like a child who's learning the names of objects or wild animals from a picture book, Billy is starting to recognize that his own emotions play a key role in effectively regulating the inputs from the paleomammalian cortex. Now, it's time to integrate the emotions associated with his *not me* experience into his identity.

Once he's fluent in these simple exercises, we slowly begin to peel back the layers of his emotional dissociation caused by the death of his friends. This allows him to experience the feelings he's suppressed for many years. Because of the association of "not me" emotions combined with intense anxiety, this is a difficult period for him often filled with frequent outbursts of anger, rage, grief, and tears. Over time, though, he is able to bridge the gap between his emotions and actions and recognizes that not only are they a part of *him* but they're also a part of being human.

As his emotional understanding and acceptance grows, I'm able to focus on helping him to manage his chronic stress. During this phase of his treatment, we repeatedly discuss his experiences in Vietnam at deeper psychological levels, and he begins to release his attachment to the guilt that has tortured him. This allows him to reconnect with certain aspects of his pre-trauma identity (the *good me*) and reduces his psychological stress to manageable levels even though the ghosts of war never fully left.

❧

There's a reason why ancient texts say that the truth will set you free. Over the next three years, Billy fully commits to the therapeutic process, and his ulcers started to heal, which stops his internal bleeding. While he could never work on cars again, he was able to resume contact with his remaining family members (his father had long passed away by this point), and he also found purpose in working as a volunteer with a veteran's outreach organization, which helped him understand his own experiences and feelings.

At the time of Billy's treatment, the field's understanding of post-traumatic stress was in its infancy, and I believe my treatment approach with him would be slightly different today. Certainly, it would include the use of psychotropic medications that were not available at the time, and our therapeutic conversations would involve more education on the impact of the trauma, but I would still prioritize listening and exploring his experience, which is a key element in any effective psychotherapy.

Treating Billy had a profound effect on me in my journey toward becoming a psychotherapist. He was my first long-term patient, and working with him taught me many lessons, the most important of which being that there's an emotional price to pay for the therapist. In guiding the patient out of their own labyrinth of suffering, one often dances with them along the razor's edge between sanity and madness.

This experience also taught me that psychotherapy is not a church or courtroom. It is not a place for moral judgments of guilt or innocence. Rather, it is a sacred space of transcendence and reconciliation beyond the mental defenses designed to keep us safe. However, it can sometimes entrap the doctor, and he or she must confront their own dark thoughts, actions, and emotions for treatment to be effective for the patient. For Billy, the therapeutic space is where he finally chose to untangle the ropes of death and murder that were strangling him. It is also the space where I not only shared his experience but absorbed them, and in doing so became changed somewhat like the *sin-eaters* of my Irish ancestors.

Questions for Consideration

1. Do you agree with the author's modern-day evaluation of how he would treat patients now versus how he treated him in the past? What would you do differently?
2. If you agreed with the author's handling of Billy's situation, why does this story resonate with you?
3. Tell a story of someone you helped who may have experienced a similar situation. What worked and what didn't? How did you evaluate them?
4. How do you think in-person consultations affected Billy? Do you believe he could have been treated effectively via an online therapy?
5. When does guilt serve as a healthy motivator for growth, and when does it become destructive to one's mental well-being?
6. In your opinion, how can a therapist help a patient transform guilt into accountability and self-compassion?
7. From your perspective, is it possible to completely separate one's emotions from the person they're helping—or should the goal be to incorporate them in the therapeutic process? If so, how?
8. How do you think trauma can impact one's sense of self both neurologically and psychologically?

THE DENTAL PATIENT

**VA Medical Center
Newington, Connecticut, 1982**

THE WAITING ROOM IS PACKED, and the doctors and the medical staff are caught up in a whirlwind of crises, cases, and care due to the waves of Vietnam vets flooding into the system. I'm swamped in my new role as a crisis consultant to the mental hygiene clinic at the Newington VA hospital, and even though it is my second week in the position, I'm still trying to figure out exactly what I do.

What I do know is that the crisis consultant, or, as everyone else calls it the "Friday consultant", is a new function at the clinic that was created at the end of my internship. While its primary purpose is to help reduce the workload of the clinical staff on Fridays, it also supports my research at the university on relapse in the treatment of alcoholism.

As I shuffle through the paperwork of inpatients, my office telephone rings. Placing the receiver against my ear, I hear a distressed male voice.

"Come quick! There is an emergency in the dental clinic!" he whispers loudly.

I'm puzzled since dental clinics aren't known for having *psychiatric* emergencies, so I reply half joking, "You know this is the mental health clinic, right?"

Apparently, this is not the time for sarcasm, as I hear the fear in his voice intensify.

"Yes, yes! Mental health, I know! Please come quickly! It's one of our patients, and everybody is scared."

I hang up the phone, rush out my office and sprint down the stairs toward the dental clinic. When I reach the bottom of the stairwell and push through the doors, I can see that something is terribly wrong.

The layout of this particular dental facility at the VA is flimsy at best. It's a wide-open space at the end of a corridor that's subdivided into small cubicles which contain various dental equipment and chairs each enclosed by a thin cloth of curtains on runners hung from the ceiling. It reminds me of pictures of hastily built military field hospitals. However, this isn't my first concern. When I look around the room, the entire clinic staff of dentists, nurses, and technicians are standing with their backs pressed against the walls, terrified.

Seeing me, the chief dentist, a short, balding, and heavyset man with thick plastic-rimmed glasses dressed in a white lab coat, rushes over. Sweating and breathing heavily, he wipes his brow and points to one of the cubicles.

"He's in there," he says, trembling.

I steady my gaze and wait until he slows his breathing.

"What seems to be the problem, Doctor?" I ask.

Still pointing at the cubicle, he replies, "The patient in there is demanding to have his dentures fixed, and he is very upset."

The emergency suddenly doesn't feel like a crisis anymore. Rather, it seems that the VA bureaucracy has gone mad for leaving me to deal with a dentist who doesn't want to fix dentures on a Friday afternoon, especially when there are so many new patients that I need to admit and not enough beds.

In the most reassuring tone I can muster, I answer, "Well, why don't you just fix his dentures?"

His eyes grow wide-eyed and desperate. "Because he doesn't *have* any dentures."

The *aha!* moment sinking, I realize that there really is a psychiatric emergency.

"Oh. I see," I say sheepishly. "What is his name?"

"He says his name is Manny[1]. He told us he is from the VA in Puerto Rico."

Cautiously approaching the cubicle, I notice that Manny is a short and attractive young man in his twenties. He is pacing rapidly around the room, and his eyes dart from me to the staff who stare at him in fear. I sit down in a plastic chair at the edge of the space to avoid scaring him.

After motioning for him to sit, I introduce myself.

"Hi, Manny. My name is Bob. I'm from the mental hygiene

---

1. Name has been changed.

clinic, and I am here to help you. What seems to be the problem?"

His hands and legs are shaking uncontrollably as he sits down. I have seen these involuntary movements before with other patients. He's clearly agitated.

"I need to have my dentures fixed, please!" he begs, the desperation in his voice fully palpable.

Taking a deep, slow breath, I reply, "Manny, the doctors here tell me that you don't have any dentures, so they can't fix them."

He stops fidgeting, but I can see the sweat dripping off his forehead. Fear is consuming him.

"Somebody has to do something 'cause my teeth are talking to me, and I can't stand it! I want it to stop!"

"Oh, I see. Well, let's you and I go to my office, so I can see about getting that problem fixed for you," I say calmly.

Manny nods. "You're mental hygiene, right?"

I smile, guessing that this is my new nickname for the day and say, "Yeah, Manny. I'm mental hygiene."

Reassured, Manny relaxes as I lead him to my office. The dental staff sigh in relief, letting out one synchronous exhale.

Mental hygiene...

When I was working as an intern and consultant for the VA in the early-mid 1980s, the facilities where the mental health professionals worked were called mental hygiene clinics. This label struck me as quaint and conjured up in my irreverent Monty Python mind the image of a group men in white coats dismissing patients' mental health issues with statements like Well, I know you are hallucinating and suicidally depressed, but I think if you just brush your teeth twice a day and get a good night's sleep, you will be alright. And don't forget! Good diet and exercise will do wonders for you!

Despite such thoughts, the expression "mental hygiene" is part of an American mental health movement from the early 20th century based on the ideas of the famous psychiatrist Adolf Meyer who dominated psychiatric thinking until the 1960s. Influenced by Freud's theories that emphasized the importance of early childhood experiences in psychological adjustment in adulthood, Meyer believed that most mental health illnesses were rooted in habits acquired from living in difficult neighborhoods or from being raised by unequipped and/or dysregulated parents.

He also emphasized that combating mental illness required identifying its social and environmental causes. He labeled this movement "mental hygiene" to align it with other popular progressive-era, public hygiene movements aimed at ameliorating the negative effects of industrialization, urbanization, and immigration such as the *social hygiene* movement (which attempted to reduce the spread of sexually transmitted diseases), and the *physical hygiene* movement (which taught habits of cleanliness, good nutrition, and fitness). Since many of the psychiatrists who were creating the modern VA mental health system after World War II had been a part of these changes, they adopted the term "mental hygiene" for their psychiatric clinics.

By the time I began treating Manny, the movement had largely been eclipsed by the advances in neuroscience and psychopharmacology that reshaped the understanding of mental illness in the latter part of the century. Most of the psychiatrists and psychologists that I worked with during my time with the VA were focused on medical-and science-based treatments and had long ago given up diagnoses based on philosophical speculations although there were some who were still enchanted by them.

~

As I speak with Manny in my office, an unusual story emerges. Through his fear and confusion, he shares that he's just recently flown in from Puerto Rico and is trying to solve a problem involving a motor vehicle accident with his brother's car.

"I'm from San Juan. Lived there my whole life, except when I was in the Army," he says. "I was raised by my aunt and uncle. Never met my mother or father. They told me that my mother was too ill to take care of me and that my father was away in the Army. I don't think they were married. Anyway, my *tía* and *tío*[2] eventually adopted me, but they had lots of other kids, so they didn't pay much attention to me. I never really felt like I was part of the family except for my older cousin, Jose, who always looked out for me."

"What was your relationship like with Jose?" I inquire.

"Jose was like my big brother. If I got into trouble, he would straighten it out for me. He took care of me, and I always looked up to him."

Manny then explains that after he graduated from high school, he met a spiffily dressed recruiting sergeant who convinced him that enlisting in the Army would allow him to *Be all that he could be.* This appealed to him since the only thing he really knew about his father was that he had been in the Army, but, as it turned out, the recruitment slogan didn't live up to Manny's expectations.

He was able to handle basic training due to his physical

---

2. *Tia*—aunt; *tio*—uncle

fitness, and he adapted well to the formation drills, but when he was waiting to be sent to advanced infantry training, he began experiencing his first serious psychiatric symptoms.

"I remember the first time I heard the voices. I was alone in the barracks. It was late afternoon, and we had just finished drill. I hear someone calling my name, but no one was there. I remember being spooked by it. It kept happening after that. I kept hearing that voice calling my name. Then, the voice began to change."

Eventually, the voice started telling him things. Things about himself. Horrible things, obscene things, frightening things. The voice also told him to do things, bad things, but he resisted. It was around this time when he first heard his teeth talking to him. He described the experience as like having a radio in his mouth that would broadcast all the terrible things that the voice would tell him to do. Then the paranoia set in. He believed that everyone around him was changing and looking at him differently. He felt they were suspicious of him. He worried that they were putting bad thoughts in his head, or worse, that they could read his mind and somehow knew about the voice and what it was telling him to do.

Frightened, he lost sleep, stopped eating, and began losing weight. Eventually, his sergeant sent him to the base hospital where he was immediately admitted and medicated. After receiving treatment, while the voices didn't completely leave, they did fade into the background of his awareness. He was then transferred to a larger Army hospital where he received a medical discharge with a diagnosis of schizophrenia and was transferred back to the VA hospital in San Juan.

Manny was an inpatient there for several months. The doctors had difficulty stabilizing him because the medications for treating schizophrenia weren't as effective as they are today. However, Manny slowly started showing signs of improvement. The hallucinations and the paranoia began to fade, but what Manny and the doctors didn't know was that his problems were about to get worse.

After speaking with him, it's clear to me that the Army and VA doctors correctly diagnosed him as suffering from schizophrenia, one of the most severe and debilitating of the psychiatric disorders.

First described clinically by the Swiss psychiatrist Eugen Bleuler in 1908, the disorder can involve an array of symptoms including auditory hallucinations (kinesthetic and visual ones are rarer) and delusional, illogical, or disordered thinking also known as a thought disorder[3]. Individuals with this disease can often display abnormal emotional expressions such as agitation or affective flattening or blunting[4], inappropriate laughing, ritualized and repetitive movements, and unusual forms of dress.

Epidemiological studies have indicated that it is a condition that affects around 1% of the world's population and is found in every country around the globe. Historical research even indicates that it existed in nomadic hunter-gatherer societies where such individuals were often revered as seers and prophets who could communicate with the supernatural. In the Middle Ages, individuals with schizophrenia were thought to be possessed by demons and were burned at the stake. In the early industrial age, they were felt to be social misfits and

---

3. Thought disorder involves eccentricities in thinking, language, and communication.

4. Affective flattening or emotional blunting or, refers to a condition where an individual experiences a significant reduction in their ability to express or feel emotions.

were jailed. It wasn't until the end of the 19th century that the disease was recognized as a medical condition and not a form of social maladjustment in need of incarceration.

Since it was first described by Bleuler, the scientific understanding and treatment of schizophrenia has significantly evolved from this bizarre and cruel history with genetic studies in the 1960s and 70s[5] clearly demonstrating that schizophrenia is inherited and has existed for as long as the modern Homo sapien brain.

The same studies, however, also demonstrated that heredity does not always equate to destiny. Even in monozygotic twins who share 100% of the same DNA, the disease only occurs 50% of the time. This observation led to the current diathesis-stress model, which posits that certain psychological disorders, such as schizophrenia, develop as a result of an underlying genetic vulnerability (*diathesis*) that only manifests when the person encounters an external stressor.

This is further demonstrated by the fact that the onset of schizophrenia usually occurs in one's late teens or early twenties and is usually associated with a transitional life experience such as entering puberty, leaving home, starting a new job, or going to college. Other events like the death of a loved one or the end of a relationship can trigger the onset as well, especially if the individual is relatively young.

Patients with this disorder are often disturbed and frightened by their symptoms. They are also subject to bouts of deep

---

5. Specifically, these studies indicated in monozygotic twins having 100% of the same DNA, one twin with the disease meant that the other would develop it 50% of the time. In dizygotic twins and siblings with 50% of the same DNA, schizophrenia occurred only about 10 to 20% of the time, and in adopted siblings with no shared DNA the rate dropped back to 1%. (Kendler, K. S., et al. (1993) and Gottesman, I. I. (1991)

depression and prone to suicidal thoughts[6]. However, some patients grow so accustomed to their symptoms that they are not disturbed by them. For example, a woman whom I treated after Manny believed that she and others could insert their thoughts into each other's minds without directly communicating with them. A form of thought disorder known as thought insertion or thought broadcasting. In our discussions, she was surprised when I told her that I did not have the same ability she had, and she commented rather morosely, "Oh, you didn't have the operation, did you?" I remember thinking, *Gee, I wish I'd had the operation* before my reality testing[7] kicked in, which is an example of how contagious delusional thinking can be.

～

San Juan, Puerto Rico, 1982

With medication and the support and structure of the inpatient unit at the VA hospital in Puerto Rico, Manny's condition gradually improved. His treatment team also felt that it would be good for him to have a half-day pass to visit with his family. His aunt and uncle expressed their enthusiasm for the idea and arranged for his cousin, Jose, to pick him up at the hospital. The visit went well, and later that day, Jose returned Manny to the hospital without incident.

---

6. The clinical literature shows that about 20 to 40% of schizophrenic patients make suicide attempts and the actual suicide rates among patients with schizophrenia spectrum disorders ranges between 5 and 13% vs. <1% for the general population. (Singh, 2018)
7. Reality testing: the ability of an individual to align their beliefs and perceptions accurately with the external world and distinguish between reality and fantasy.

Since the half-day pass was so successful, the treatment team decided to give him a full-day pass the next week so he could stay overnight. Jose once again picked him up driving his red Ford mustang, which Manny absolutely adored, and to celebrate the occasion, allowed Manny to drive from the hospital to his aunt and uncle's home as a special treat.

Unfortunately, on their way home, the main highway in San Juan alternated between frenetic highway racing and grid-lock traffic jams with drivers weaving between lanes nearly scraping any car in their way. When one speed-racing driver cut Manny off, he panicked and slammed on his brakes. Seconds later, the car behind him plowed into his cousin's red Mustang pushing them into the car that just cut him off, causing a huge pileup on the highway.

When the police arrived, people were understandably upset and looking for someone to blame. Jose remained calm, dealt with the police, and exchanged information with the other drivers. After examining his vehicle, he saw that even though the front end and trunk of the Mustang were damaged, the car was still drivable.

Manny, however, was so shaken up that he was unable to drive. Scared, he began to decompensate and felt the voices and paranoia starting to close in even though he did every-thing in his power to resist.

When Manny and Jose finally arrive at his aunt and uncle's house late that afternoon, everyone was initially upset about the accident but decided not to let it ruin Manny's planned overnight visit. Soon, dinner was served and everyone began settling down for the night.

Manny remained quiet throughout the evening, trying to control his thoughts as flashbacks of the accident over-whelmed him. Consumed by feelings of guilt over damaging Jose's car, the voices in his head grew louder and scarier, but through the fog of confusing thoughts and emotions, a detail from the accident emerged into his awareness.

Before speaking to the police, Jose had given him his insurance card to hold. Manny recalled the name on the card: *The Hartford Insurance Company.* Suddenly, through the fog of the voices and fear, Manny knew exactly what to do to fix the situation. He would go to the headquarters of the insurance company in Hartford, Connecticut and file the claim in person for the accident to have his cousin's car repaired.

Early the next morning, Manny woke up before everyone else, walked to his bank to withdraw all the money from his checking account, hailed a cab to the airport, and purchased a ticket to Kennedy Airport in New York with a connecting flight to Brainard Airport just outside of Hartford.

However, in his haste to make it to the airport, Manny forgot to bring his medication. By the time he arrived at Kennedy several hours later, the effects of his morning medications had worn off and his hallucinations returned. Increasingly disoriented, he barely made his connecting flight to Brainard.

By midafternoon when he arrived in Connecticut, the effects of his medications had completely worn off and his auditory hallucinations were so overwhelming that in the haze of the psychosis, he lost track of where he was or why he was there. After exiting the airplane, he stumbled out of the terminal and walked over to one of the taxi cabs waiting for passengers and said to the driver, "Please take me to the VA hospital."

Thankfully, the Brainard Airport, even though it is a small regional airport, serviced the state capitol, the corporate headquarters for several major insurance companies, including The Hartford, the University of Connecticut Medical School, and the VA Medical Center at Newington, so when

Manny said, "Take me to the VA," the cab driver knew exactly where to go.

The main entrance at Newington had a circular drive with a fountain in the center and a colonial portico over the entrance, which was where the cab driver dropped Manny off. When he entered the building, Manny was confronted with a great semicircular, teak and rosewood desk that was manned by pleasant and motherly woman with white hair and a gentle smile whose job was to provide information and direct patients to the appropriate clinic.

From what I determined after speaking with her, Manny had stumbled through the entrance, looking confused and disoriented.

"He seemed very upset," she said to me over the phone, "but sometimes patients are like that, so I said what I always say, 'How may I direct you?' He responded, and I must say that he was very adamant that he needed to be seen by mental health and dental. Well, I checked the spread sheet for the open appointment slots for the mental health and dental clinics and there were no scheduled openings in the mental hygiene clinic until Monday morning. However, there was an opening in the dental clinic for that afternoon, so I asked him if he would like that appointment. He mumbled something I didn't understand, as if he was talking to someone else, and then said, 'Yes, dental, please!' So, I directed him there. I must say he did seem to be a very strange fellow, but mine is not to judge."

By the time Manny wandered into the dental clinic, everything seemed alien to him. The building's set up and its entrance were different and the woman behind the desk, while pleasant, looked and spoke differently than the woman at the VA in San Juan. As soon as Manny realized that this was not his VA, his teeth started screaming at him.

~

As Manny relates his story, he seems fairly calm and lucid, but I can see that he is becoming restless and struggling to control something inside of him.

"Manny, I would like you to stay with us. I think we can help. I am going to call a friend of mine whom I trust and whom *you* can trust. Between us all, I believe we can fix your problem, okay?"

He doesn't respond to my suggestion and seems to be lost in a swirl of thoughts, which ticks up my anxiety a bit since I'm not sure what he'll do next. After a moment, he looks at me and nods.

"Okay, Mental Hygiene, okay," he says.

Standing next to him, I pick up the phone and call the psychiatric unit.

"Is Dom there? This is Bob. I need a favor."

Dr. Angelino Dominick, who likes to be called "Dom" due to his disdain for formality, believes it gets in the way of good treatment. He's also in charge of inpatient psychiatric admissions. Built like an NFL linebacker, standing just over 6'2", he has an unruly mop of black hair and a beard. He also happens to be a brilliant psychiatrist. In the past, he was an Army doctor and completed several tours of duty at Bethesda while being trained in psychiatry at John Hopkins University. He's currently doing NIMH funded research on psychotropic medications at the University's Medical School. He's also from New York City like me, which I think is partly why we're great colleagues.

Hearing the click of the phone, I say, "Dom, I have a hot one."

"Aren't they all?" he responds.

"No, this one is different. Young vet in his early twenties.

History of auditory hallucinations, paranoid, and delusional thinking. Very disoriented and frightened. He is decompensating in my office as we speak. He came here from Puerto Rico today."

After a brief pause, I add, "Also, he tells me his teeth are talking to him."

Sensing I've piqued his interest, he says, "His teeth talk to him? Hmm. I'll send a tech. We'll take care of him."

"Thanks, Dom."

I turn to Manny to tell him that Dom has agreed to admit him, but I can see that he is no longer with me. He is calmer, but it's clear that he has withdrawn into his delusions and the inner dialogue of the voices in his head.

Over the next few weeks as I adjust to the rapid pace of crisis admissions during the day and the relapse experiment at night, I don't have much time to check on Manny, but I know that he is being well cared for by Dom and his team on the inpatient unit. That is, until I receive a call from Dom.

"Bob, I want you to take another look at our boy."

Hearing the phrase 'our boy' makes me think that Dom apparently has decided to take Manny under his wing, which, all things considered, doesn't strike me as a bad option for Manny.

"I think he's better," Dom continues. "But since you saw him before, I'd like your opinion as a comparison."

"Be glad to, Dom."

Manny comes to my office the next day unescorted and dressed in hospital pajamas, a thin robe, and slippers. He makes himself comfortable in the chair reserved for my patients as I sit at my desk. He looks much less haunted than the last time I saw him, and it's apparent that he has gained some weight. I also can't help but notice that there's an undeniable spark in his eyes.

"Hi, Mental Hygiene," he says.

I smile and nod. "How's it going, Manny?"

"Great! This is the best VA I have ever been in. I like the people here and Dr. Dom's cool."

"That's good. I think he's cool, too," I reply, matching his upbeat tone.

"Yeah, they even told me about my vocational and educational benefits and that I can train for a job."

At this point, I am impressed with both the change in his demeanor and his musings. He's relaxed and no longer frightened by the sound of unfamiliar voices.

Following his train of thought, I decide to test the limits of his recovery.

"What kind of job would you like?"

"I'm going to get trained to be an airline pilot," he says.

I'm a little taken back by his response. It's not bizarre like the day we met when he thought his teeth were talking to him, but it is unrealistic given his psychiatric history. Up until now, the logic of his thought processes has improved, so it's possible that this may just be a naïve thought and not the result of his delusions, so I decide to explore his thinking further.

"Manny, don't you think that you having had several psychiatric hospitalizations might count against you when you apply?"

He responds with a mischievous smile, "Not, if I don't tell 'em."

Stunned, I briefly fixate on the fact that no one would know otherwise. Psychiatric records are very confidential and the disturbing thought of being a passenger on a plane flown by Captain Manny crosses my mind until he adds, "And if my teeth don't talk, I'll be okay."

While this statement relieves my Captain Manny fantasy, it also reminds me that schizophrenia is a chronic episodic disease and that, while Manny is definitely better, he is not yet stable and may never be. His psychotic thought processes still linger just beneath the surface and can intensify under stressful conditions. This provides me the information I need to complete the assessment Dom asked for, and I decide to end the interview.

"Okay by you if I give Dom a call about our conversation and let him know how you are doing?"

"Okay by me, Mental Hygiene."

I send Manny back to the psychiatric ward and call Dom to let him know what has transpired.

"Oh. I see...Hmm. Thanks, Bob," he says somewhat disappointed by my report.

In the VA system, the type of hospital I work at is seen as an acute care facility with some rehabilitation capacity and a wide range of outpatient services. Inpatient stays are supposed to be relatively short—a few days in most cases, maybe a week if the situation is particularly severe. However, if patients are in need of extended treatment, they may be transferred to one of the long-term care hospitals in the VA system.

Nevertheless, Dom has a habit of stretching the length of hospitalization for his patients. While he sometimes takes heat from the hospital administration, given his reputation, they generally don't press him too much. In Manny's case, Dom has really stretched it, allowing him to stay at our facility for three months, well beyond the standard operating procedures. I can't help but admire Dom's commitment to his patients and his soft spot for Manny, but I guess even he has his limits.

Manny's situation is also complicated politically because our attempts to transfer him back to the VA in Puerto Rico have been rejected cold. Apparently, Manny's elopement to Connecticut while on a full-day pass was the scandal of the century for them and caused a full-scale investigation, which led to several staff members being removed. According to Dom, the San Juan hospital has zero interest in readmitting Manny, and, sadly, even his own family doesn't want to see him.

My initial reaction to this news is anger. *Bureaucrats covering their asses.* Having worked for the feds, I've seen this kind of behavior before. In fact, one of my reasons for leaving the agency was to get away from all the red tape, so being confronted with the same levels of bureaucratic nonsense in the medical field not only causes my anger to boil but increases my commitment to protect my patients from it.

"Bob, I think we are going to have to transfer our boy." I can hear the frustration and worry in his voice. "While he is better, there are still the breakthrough hallucinations, and he still has the delusion about his teeth talking to him. I can't discharge him to the street, but I can't hold on to him any longer either."

"It's interesting. Manny has a girlfriend of sorts up here. Her name is Elena[8]. It's weird. She has a similar diagnosis of schizophrenia, but, get this, she gets into an accident in Miami on the I-95 and then flies to Hartford because her insurance, just like with Manny's cousin, is with The Hartford Insurance Company, and she wants to file the claim in person. What are the odds of the two of them being on the same psychiatric unit at the same time? They seem to get along and have a calming

____

8. Name has been changed.

effect on each other. Anyway, administration says that we need to transfer both of them, and I want you to make the arrangements."

As my anger fades, I remember a conversation I had during clinical supervision with Dr. Daniels the week prior. Anticipating that administration might pull the plug on Manny's stay at Newington, Dr. Daniels tried to prepare me mentally for what's to come.

"It seems that Manny is making some progress here, but it's slow. You know he can't stay here forever, though, Bob. Since Puerto Rico won't take him back, he will have to go to long-term care here in the States."

With visions of large warehouse-like facilities unable to provide personalized care for Manny, I slump back into my chair feeling frustrated and defeated.

"Bob, you know there are excellent long-term care facilities within our system that have specialized care units for schizophrenia. In fact, there is one which is not far from here in Montrose, New York. It's about 75 miles away. Some of my other patients have done well there, and based on everything you've told me about Manny, I think it could be a good fit for him when he has to be discharged."

Twirling my pen, I decide to float an idea to Dom.

"What if Manny and Elena went to the long-term care facility at Montrose?"

"That's a great idea!" Dom exclaims. "I don't know why I didn't think of it. I'll write up the paperwork."

"Send it to me, and I'll take care of the details," I say, feeling pleased. "Also, one more thing. I'd like to see Manny before he goes."

"No problem. I'll set up a time for you on the unit."

Dom sends the paperwork for the transfer later that day, and I contact the admissions department at Montrose. The social worker thankfully cooperates, and we make arrangements for their transportation. When everything is ready, I buzz onto the inpatient unit to meet with Manny early that next morning. However, before I talk to Manny, Dom pulls me aside with an air of practiced nonchalance.

"Would you like to meet his girlfriend?" he asks, smiling.

"Yes," I say, curious about their relationship.

Dom leads me to a common area on the unit. Sitting at one of the tables is a young woman who appears to be in her twenties with a thin build and long blonde hair.

As we approach, Dom begins to make the introductions. "Elena, I would like you to meet—"

"Oh, you're Mental Hygiene! Manny's told me all about you!"

She invites me to sit with her, folding her arms across her lap.

"I was pretty confused when I first got here," she says. "The voices were so loud and kept telling me to do things, but Dr. Dom has really helped me with that. They're not so loud now, and meeting Manny has helped, too."

"How are things going with him?" I inquire.

"Well, I think he's kind of cute, and he's easy for me to talk to. The staff here are nice. Not like in some hospitals that I've been in, but it can get kind of lonely, especially in the evening when there's not much going on."

As Elena shares more about her experience, I am curious about whether Manny's delusions have come up and how she deals with them in their relationship.

"Elena, has Manny ever talked about his teeth?"

"Oh sure. He's bothered by them sometimes, but, you know, that's just part of who Manny is. I'm not bothered by it. Heck, I've got my own stuff, but none of it gets in the way when we are talking to each other. I think that's why I like him. We seem to be able to accept each other."

Struck by her basic human need for intimacy—to be seen, understood, and accepted by another—, I realize that she's describing Sullivan's wisdom all over again: *We are all more simply human than otherwise.*

I leave to find Manny, who, by the time I knock on his door, is already packing. He's dressed in a brand-new outfit made up of dark denim jeans, a short sleeved T-shirt, and sneakers—a nice contrast from the usual hospital apparel.

As I enter the room, he smiles and greets me with the same introduction that I know I'll miss.

"Hi, Mental Hygiene."

"Hi, Manny," I reply.

He sits on the bed and motions me toward the only chair in the room.

"So, I hear you will be leaving soon," I say.

"Yeah, going to the hospital over at Montrose. Don't know much about the place," he replies.

"I hear it's very good. Nice place, and the staff are like here. I think they can help you, like we did."

"You know, it's the teeth. Just couldn't get them to stop talking, but it's a little better."

"Well, I think the folks at Montrose can keep working with you on that problem, and it may continue to get better. Not get in the way so much."

"Sure hope so 'cause they've caused me a lot of trouble in the past," he says, lowering his head.

Sensing that he doesn't want to talk about his teeth anymore, I change the topic.

"Dom told me about you and Elena. I just met her. She seems nice."

"Yeah, she's like me. We get along. I am able to talk with her and, you know, when I am with her, my teeth don't talk so much. Also, she's going to Montrose, too, so, we can still be together."

"That's good, Manny."

"Yeah, it is," he says.

We both pause, soaking up the last moments of our final conversation together. Then, Manny reaches out and shakes my hand with a smirk.

"Well, see you around, Mental Hygiene."

"See you around, Manny."

"And, Mental Hygiene?"

"Yes, Manny?"

"Thanks."

~

At midday, the medical transport takes Manny and Elena to Montrose. The drive is about 90 minutes, and as I assess another patient for admission, I find myself contemplating how Manny and Elena are handling their new hospital. That is, until I receive a call from the chief psychiatrist at Montrose who's irate.

Shouting into the phone, she says, "What were you thinking sending this guy to us? Do you know the kind of patients we deal with here? The woman's okay for this type of facility, but the guy is too sane. A little scared maybe, but he doesn't belong here."

I remain quiet as she rages on about how Manny is not the type of patient that should be at her hospital. When she finally pauses to take a breath, I quickly interject.

"Look, maybe you are right and maybe I've made a mistake. I can arrange for him to be brought back to us, but before I do, I'd like you to check something out. I'd like you to ask him about his teeth."

She huffs in frustration and hangs up the phone.

I return to patient admissions when suddenly my phone rings 10 minutes later.

The same voice is now apologetic.

"Oh, yes, he'll fit in nicely here," she says. "Sorry about the mix up."

"No problem," I say, returning to the inpatient admission form.

I lost track of Manny after his transfer to Montrose, but I like to imagine him living a happier, quieter life with Elena by his side. People do better when they are not alone.

Humans, after all, are a pack species by nature, and we need intimacy from other humans not just to survive but to thrive. Moreover, the symptoms of any human pathology tend to improve when someone has a person—or better yet, a community—with whom to share the experience.

Much has significantly improved in the psychiatric treatment of schizophrenia since I treated Manny. In particular, the medications we use are more effective in controlling the acute symptoms of the disorder and the psychotherapeutic approaches are more psychoeducational[9], teaching coping skills as opposed to searching for the root developmental cause —the schizophrenogenic mother. While medication combined

---

9. Psychoeducation is a therapeutic approach in which the patient is provided knowledge, information, resources, and coping skills related to their specific mental health condition or concern.

with psychotherapy and a sense of community are still necessary components of effective treatment, neither is a cure.

As I learned from working with Manny, severe psychiatric disorders like schizophrenia do not just affect the individual's psychological and emotional functioning; they also affect their humanity by creating social isolation, alienation, loss of community, and the ancillary problems of poverty, homelessness, drug use and poor health care—all of which exacerbate the patient's condition. These are challenges that everyone witnesses on the streets, but collectively society struggles to meet, or even at times acknowledge them, choosing rather to avert their eyes or worse blame the victim.

Questions for Consideration

1. Does the word "hygiene" minimize the severity of the situation Manny was dealing with? Was the term too broad-stroked to accurately convey his disorder? Could there have been better terminology at the time? How do labels impact patient treatment? How has modern terminology evolved from this?
2. Why do you think that the author initially felt confused when he went to the dental clinic? What could have been done or said differently to provide clarity to the author, so he knew what he was getting into?
3. How did Manny get past airport security while dealing with this type of episode? Do you think modern protocols would be able identify and quickly address a challenge such as this?

4. The author imagined Manny and Elena coping together. What do you think would have happened to Manny if Elena got better and left the hospital or was transferred elsewhere?

5. Do you think that Manny's family abandoned Manny? Do you think they would ever reconnect if Manny was in a better place mentally?

6. Why would hospital administration have protocols that would cause a patient like Manny to be potentially discharged? What would have happened if they were both discharged from the hospital on an outpatient basis? What would have happened if Montrose hospital wasn't available? What other options would have been available at the time, and would they have been worse? Would Manny in some way have been forgotten?

7. Why do you think Dr. Dom took a special interest in Manny's case? Why did he appear to have an over-the-top trust in the author who was just an intern? Did he see a special talent or skill in the author? What would be a normal trust level for an intern? What skills did he see in the author?

8. Why are there such varying degrees of treatment at other hospitals with similar patients? Is it staffing? Training? Are some people just not in the right field? Are hospitals getting too many difficult patients? Would Manny have been more challenging if he hadn't met Elena? Do you believe that the author and Dom's humanity toward Manny helped in his treatment? How does humanity impact treatment and treatment impact humanity?

THE DESIGNER DRUG

PATIENTS WHO ARE ABUSING substances tend to be behaviorally unstable. A New York City burglary detective who I worked with once observed, "If I come to the scene of a burglary and the lock on the door has been picked, I know I am dealing with a professional burglar, but if the door has been ripped off its hinges, then I am dealing with a drug addict.

VA Medical Center
Newington, Connecticut, 1983

The rest of the staff have gone home for the weekend, and the clinic is quiet. I'm alone at my desk finishing the paper work from the day's admissions.

Leaning back in my chair, I take a deep breath and realize that I feel tired both physically and emotionally. It's the end of my first year as the *Friday consultant,* and it's been a long day with several crisis admissions. However, I'm in a particularly good mood since my wife, Astrid, and I are about to go on a long overdue vacation for ten days to her family's beach house in Yabucoa, Puerto Rico, a remarkably beautiful and peaceful place on the Caribbean side of the island where we were married. It's a much-needed break from the stress of the consulting duties and the research I'm conducting for my dissertation, which requires monthly trips between Connecticut and New York City.

As I put the last of my papers into a shoulder bag, my fantasies of palm trees, white sandy beaches, and the warm Caribbean Ocean are suddenly interrupted by my phone. Giving a long exhale, I pick it up.

"Gillespie, Mental Hygiene Clinic," I answer wearily.

"Help me! Help me!" a voice shouts, immediately yanking me out of both my fatigue and my beach reverie.

"Who is this?" I ask.

"It's me, Henry[1], and you've got to help me!"

"Henry what's the matter?" I ask, recognizing his name and voice as a patient I treated when I was an intern.

"I'm stuck in this phone booth, and I can't get out!"

The panic in his voice reverberates through the phone, and I can hear the tightness in his breath. My mind immediately jumps into emergency-response mode. *First, I have to calm him down. Then, I need to find out where he's located so I can call 911*

---

1. Name has been changed.

and have someone take him to the hospital. However, as I am composing this plan, I can also hear my wife's voice in the back of my mind reminding me that we have to be on time to catch the red-eye to San Juan.

"Henry, I want you to take a deep breath and then slowly let it out, okay?" I say, adjusting my shoulder bag strap on my shoulder.

"You don't understand! I can't breathe! I have been in this fucking phone booth for 45 minutes, and I can't open the doors!"

Sounds of the rattling phone booth doors echo through the phone.

During panic, the paleomammalian cortex hijacks the neocortex and the body is flooded with adrenalin. The body's heart rate and breathing increase rapidly, and visual focus narrows to only the immediate surroundings. All logical thinking and reasoning cease, and survival mode kicks in, making decisions impulsive and immediate. Recognizing that this is the state which Henry is in, it's time for Plan B.

"Henry, tell me where you are so I can send someone to help."

Suddenly, there is an eerie silence on the phone. I press the phone against my ear in hopes that I'll be able to decipher what's happening, but the only thing I can make out is what sounds like a body hitting the ground.

"Henry! Henry! Can you hear me? Speak to me!"

There's no reply except for the ominous sound of the dangling telephone receiver thumping against the glass of the phone booth and a symphony of cars and footsteps in the background.

Suddenly, I hear the unfamiliar voice of a bystander.

"Hey! Look at the guy with his feet sticking out of the phone booth!"

"Someone pick up the phone!" I shout, but no one seems to hear me.

With the phone pressed against my ear, I pace around my office trying to assess the situation. Henry is possibly dying, and I don't have the faintest idea of his location. Worse, I have an open phone line with no one on the other end, and, adding to my sense of urgency, is imagining Astrid waiting for me at the house with our bags packed.

As my own paleomammalian brain kicks in, thoughts of Henry in danger make difficult to come up with a logical plan.

I try to clear my head and I force myself to take a few deep breaths when a miracle happens—someone picks up the phone.

"Hello? This is Jake from J&L Ambulance. Who am I speaking with?"

"Thank God!" I shout, fully convinced of the existence of a benign divine presence in the universe.

"I'm Dr. Gillespie with the VA hospital, and the man in the phone booth's name is Henry. He's a patient. Please bring him to the ER at the hospital, and I will meet you there!"

"Oh, no! Absolutely not! We know Henry." He snarls. "The last time we tried to help him, he busted up the ambulance. No way we're taking him. No way!"

My newly found belief in divine providence begins to fade when Jake denies my request.

Trying to control my panic, I soldier on with the recalcitrant ambulance driver. Well, actually, I just start begging. Jake grows bored with my pleas, hands the phone to his partner, Linda, who apparently is the "L" in J&L Ambulance.

The exact details of our conversation aren't clear to me as I'm now experiencing a secondary wave of panic due to the adrenalin rush[2]. What promises I made to her, I do not remember. I only know that she eventually agrees to transport Henry to our ER entrance.

Calmer now that Henry is enroute, I call the ER. I don't want to take any chances with his admission, so I dash from my office to the ER where he arrives 20 minutes later, unconscious.

The ER staff take over immediately for Jake and Linda, whom I thank profusely for their help. With choreographed efficiency, they transfer him from the ambulance to the hospital gurney and whisk him into an ER treatment room. I stand by and watch as they remove his clothes and perform a cursory physical examination for wounds or injuries. As they start a saline IV, I breathe a sigh of relief.

A few minutes later an ER physician whom I know from my crisis admissions work comes out of the treatment room.

"What's his status?" I ask, pulling him to the side.

"His breathing and heart rate are regular," he responds tersely. "And his vitals are stable. It doesn't look like a heart attack or stroke. I think it's some kind of drug overdose."

I nod.

"Any idea what he took?" he asks, finally recognizing me.

"No, but he has a history of using street drugs and alcohol."

"Well, we'll take a blood sample, which should tell us what it was. I don't think he is in any immediate danger, but we'll monitor him for a while and then admit him to the acute medical unit. He'll eventually be on the psychiatric unit in Dr. Jaffe's substance abuse program. There's nothing more you can do here. I'll keep you posted."

---

2. An adrenaline rush is a physiological response triggered by the release of adrenaline (epinephrine) into the bloodstream. This response prepares the body for a "fight or flight" reaction in stressful or exciting situations. It can cause various cognitive effects that can enhance or impair mental functioning.

"Thanks. I'll be away for a few days, so please let Dr. Daniels know the updates."

"Sure, no problem."

With Henry in good hands, I drive back to the office, dashing up two flights of stairs to write up the clinical documentation for Henry's admission and leave a brief note on Dr. Daniel's desk. Afterward, I rush home where I find my wife Astrid waiting with our bags. I give her a peck on the cheek and apologize for being late. We catch our flight to San Juan with only minutes to spare. My faith in the divine now fully restored.

Henry had initially been referred to me for outpatient psychotherapy and substance abuse treatment when I was an intern. He had just completed an inpatient substance abuse treatment program designed by Dr. Jerome Jaffe[3], who was the first White House drug czar under President Nixon in the early 70s and is known for his work on opiate addiction with Vietnam veterans. The inpatient program he created at Newington was part of a joint treatment research program between the VA and the Alcohol Research Center (ARC) at the University of Connecticut Medical School where I was conducting the experiment on relapse. Our paths never crossed until Henry's admission.

As a soldier from the Korean War, Henry was older than most of the Vietnam veterans I treated as an intern. He also

---

3. In the early 1980s, Dr. Jaffe, charismatic and brilliant, was well known in the medical community for his work on addiction. He had been instrumental in working with Congress to create the National Institute on Alcohol Abuse and Alcoholism (NIAAA) that funded research at the Alcohol Research Center (ARC).

had quite a reputation among the local police and first responders in Hartford. As one seasoned nurse at the clinic told me, "Henry has been raising hell around here ever since he got back from Korea. Gets drunk and drugged up. Particularly nasty if he gets Xanax and booze. Then he likes to start a fight in some bar, gets busted up, and ends up here."

During my internship, my first impression of Henry was that while he seemed to enjoy talking with me, our conversations were having a negligible impact on his substance abuse. I did learn, however, that his experience in Korea haunted him with memories of human wave assaults[4]. He lived in New Britain, Connecticut (the home of Stanley tools) with an adult son, who was a member of a local chapter of the Outlaws Motorcycle Club. According to the nurse, the two drank and used drugs together, which frequently led to fights that required the intervention of local police.

Puerto Rico has done me some good. Tanned, relaxed, and re-energized, I walk through the doors of the Mental Hygiene clinic ready to resume the Friday consulting work. That is, until the clinic secretary informs me that Dr. Jaffe wants to see me.

---

4.   Human wave assaults were a military tactic used by the Chinese during the Korean War in which masses of their soldiers, often armed only with hand grenades, would charge at well defended South Korean and American positions. Suffering huge losses, they would use sheer numbers to overwhelm the defenders. Veterans who experienced this tactic described it as almost medieval, brutal and to hand combat. This tactic was so effective that it reversed the momentum of the war thwarting a U.S. victory in Korea which in turn, was a one of the factors that helped trigger the subsequent Cold War arms race.

"It's about that patient you admitted just before you left," she says, clearing her throat.

"Henry?"

"Yes."

"Oh no! Has he torn the place up?"

"I don't know. They just told me Dr. Jaffe wanted to see you as soon as you got back."

To say that I am a little nervous about having a meeting with the former White House drug czar under these circumstances is an understatement. My mind and heart race as I mentally prepare myself to explain what happened the evening that Henry was admitted.

Trying to keep calm, I head up to Dr. Jaffe's locked substance abuse unit. The door buzzes for me to come in, and, still fearing the worst, I see him speaking rather intensely to one of the unit's nurses in a small office reserved for the doctors near the nursing station. I knock on the open office door, and they abruptly end their conversation. The nurse quickly leaves without a word as Dr. Jaffe's eyes turn to me. *Oh my god! Were they talking about me? What have I done? What has Henry done? I'm doomed!*

Dressed in the traditional white lab coat, Dr. Jaffe is a stout man of average height in his early fifties. Balding with a fringe of white hair, a well-trimmed beard and wearing wire rimmed glasses, he is not physically imposing, but the way he carries himself conveys a sense of power and charisma that does nothing to alleviate my anxiety.

As I approach, he looks at me and smiles warmly.

"Hi, I'm Dr. Jaffe. You must be Gillespie, the consultant who admitted the patient who's been puzzling us for two weeks."

I exhale, relieved by his friendliness.

"Yes. I admitted him."

"Good. Come with me. I want you to look at him."

The sense of impending doom I feel evaporates as I realize that this is not going to be a summary execution but rather a chance to collaborate with a renowned specialist on substance abuse.

Dr. Jaffe leads me to a room on the unit that's used to keep agitated patients safe. With fittings on both the walls and floor to secure large soft cloth pads, it is consistent with my mental image of what a classic padded cell is supposed to look like according to Hollywood films. Years later, when I was directing an inpatient program in Minnesota that dealt with violent brain-injured patients, I discovered what a real padded cell should be. According to the national consultant we hired to build it, there shouldn't be any cloth padding but rather a high-tech soft polymer coating because patients could eat the fabric and die. This room, however, is not designed for patients with violent, aggressive, or suicidal behaviors. It's meant to prevent patients who are experiencing severe physical drug withdrawal symptoms, such as muscle spasms, from injuring themselves.

The space also has an observation room with a one-way mirror built into one of the walls, and this is where Dr. Jaffe leads me. When I look through the glass, I see Henry who appears unable to stand. As he crawls along the floor, he swivels and shakes his head from side to side, his vacant eyes searching longingly for something that isn't there.

"He has been like this since they brought him to the unit," Dr. Jaffe comments. "He can't stand without assistance. Hasn't said more than a few words, and they don't make much sense. Doesn't respond to questions or even simple commands either."

"Can I go in and try to talk with him?"

"That's why I asked for you. I was told you treated him

before this episode, and that he not only knows you, but had a good enough relationship with you that he called you for help. Maybe you can get through to him."

I stand by the wall next to the door for a moment and watch Henry before entering the room. I'm shocked by his condition. He looks different than when I treated him as an intern. Dressed in hospital pajamas, he looks both disheveled and disoriented as he crawls the room on his hands and knees. He stops occasionally, as if trying to orient himself but inevitably resumes his aimless journey. Having completed my observation, I enter the space, and, because there are no chairs, I squat down to be at eye level with him.

"Henry, it's me Bob. Do you remember me? I used to treat you at the clinic. You called me a couple of weeks ago when you were in trouble, remember?"

For a moment, Henry stops crawling and looks at me. I see a transient flicker of recognition in his gaze and immediately feel a surge of hope. If he recognizes me, then maybe the power of the therapeutic relationship we established during his treatment will break through to him.

"Where am I? Am I standing? I think I'm standing. Am I standing? Where am I?" He asks completely disoriented and confused.

He speaks in the same desperate voice as when he was in the phonebooth, but now I can also see the fear in his eyes. *He's disoriented. If I can help him understand where he is, it will reduce the fear and help bring him out of his confusion.*

"Henry, you are in the VA hospital," I say using the calmest tone I can muster.

But before I can even finish my sentence, Henry's recognition of me has faded. His eyes lose their focus and his gaze drifts away as he begins his restless crawling around the room once again. Trying to regain his attention, I raise my voice slightly, deepen my tone, and repeat several times, "Henry. Look at me. Look at me, Henry," but without success.

I sit quietly, watching him for a few more minutes in hopes that the recognition I saw in his eyes might return. I get up and take one more look at him before stepping out of the room and closing the door. I try to control the feeling of profound sadness welling up in me.

Dr. Jaffe, who is feverishly writing notes about the encounter, stops and, chart still in hand, approaches me in front of the two-way mirror.

"That's the way he has been since he woke up after being admitted. When he is awake, he crawls around like that all day muttering. I'm not quite sure what is going on, but thanks for trying. I will keep you posted about any developments."

"Thanks, Dr. Jaffe. Sorry, I couldn't help."

I leave the unit stunned by the change in the man I had spent hours conversing with in psychotherapy as an intern. Yes, it's true that he had a wild streak and a taste for alcohol and drugs, but he could also be insightful about himself and the world. He also brought a sly, infectious sense of humor to our work that made us both laugh at times. Seeing him like this is painfully distressing to me. *What could have reduced someone who just a year ago could carry on wide-ranging conversations to this state? What exactly happened to him?*

The following week, I stop by the unit to check on his progress. The clinicians inform me that there has been no change, and my concern escalates as his condition continues to stump even the experts.

"Bob, I'd like you to come up to the substance abuse unit this morning. We are going to try something with Henry, and I want you to participate."

I jump at the offer, immediately putting my notes on my desk.

"Absolutely! Be glad to, Dr. Jaffe."

When I arrive, I can sense a notable change in the unit's normal daily activity. The noisy murmur of background activity has ceased and everyone on the unit is focused on a patient room. Dr. Jaffe stands just down the hall conferring with a small group of nurses, doctors, and technicians.

Seeing me, he motions for me to join him and the other medical staff. The others make room for me.

"I think I might know what is wrong with Henry. I believe he is suffering from a form of delirium[5] from a drug he took. I don't know what the drug is. The drug screens from his tests were negative except for traces of marijuana, and that's not causing his condition. I speculate that someone gave him a *designer drug*[6]."

"A designer drug?" I ask, confused.

"These are not like any of the drugs that we typically encounter in our patients, and we don't know a lot about them. It's cooked up by someone in a lab to avoid detection by our tests, and, as a result, they can sometimes have weird and

---

5. Delirium is an acute mental disturbance characterized by confusion accompanied by disordered consciousness, thinking, cognition (especially attention), behavior, and hallucinations.

6. A "designer drug" is a controlled substance (i.e., drugs like stimulants, sedatives, dissociatives, cannabinoids, and psychedelics, which are regulated by federal government based on their known risk for misuse and dependence) that has been pharmaceutically manipulated to avoid classification as illegal and/or detection in standard drug tests while retaining, or in some cases enhancing, the original effects of the drug. Designer drugs emerged in the 1980s in response to the intensification of drug enforcement efforts begun a "War on Drugs" in the 1970s and were devised to circumvent new drug laws.

unpredictable effects. They've been showing up on college campuses lately and are also associated with some of the West Coast biker gangs."

Designer drug. Suddenly, I realize that I may know what happened to Henry. However, I will have to wait for him to wake up to confirm if my suspicions are right.

Dr. Jaffe continues. "If I am correct, and this is delirium, there is a way to bring him out of it, at least briefly. We are going to administer a sodium pentothal drip."

Sodium pentothal. That's truth serum! Images of spies being interrogated in Hollywood war movies suddenly flash through my mind. *How is this going to work?*

As if reading my mind, Dr. Jaffe explains, "If it is delirium, after a few drops, he should come out of it. The procedure is to administer the pentothal one drip at a time. After each drip, we will ask him some orientation questions."

He then turns and looks directly at me.

"Here's where you come in, Bob. Since he knew you before taking the drug, if he responds to the orientation questions correctly, then I want you to talk with him. If he recognizes you, it is a good indication that his symptoms are not the result of brain damage and that his memory is still intact. Later we can test his cognitive functioning more formally, but this will be a good preliminary indicator. You okay to do this?"

"Absolutely! Anything I can do to help," I exclaim, glad to be able to finally do something for Henry. The aspiring clinician in me is also intrigued by the opportunity to participate in such a unique procedure and the insights it will give me about substance abuse and the neuropsychology of Henry's condition.

Dr. Jaffe then leads me into the room where Henry is lying awake but unresponsive. His eyes no longer dart restlessly around the room but remain fixed on the ceiling. Next to the hospital bed is an IV apparatus with a clear bag marked sodium pentothal and a tape recorder on the bedside table. One of the nurses will operate the drip and the other will monitor Henry's vitals while recording. The first physician will time the procedure with a stopwatch. The other will ready himself for any emergency medical intervention should something go wrong. The two behavioral techs are there in case Henry becomes agitated. I stand opposite Henry ready to be a friendly face should he wake up.

Once everyone is in their assigned positions, Dr. Jaffe nods to the nurse with the tape recorder.

"Here we go, everyone. Drop number one."

The the clamp on the line coming from the bag of sodium pentothal opens, and the first bead enters the drop chamber and disappears down the IV line connected to Henry. The nurse notes the time and his vitals while the physician standing next to Dr. Jaffe starts his stopwatch.

Everyone in the room holds their breath.

"Henry, can you hear me? Do you know where you are?" Dr. Jaffe asks, standing over him.

Henry eyes remain fixated on the ceiling.

"Henry, can you hear me? Do you know where you are?" He repeats, unphased. "Okay, team let's administer another dose."

The physician resets his stopwatch.

"Okay, everyone. Drop two."

The same procedure continues three more times without any response from Henry. While Dr. Jaffe and his team methodically repeat the process, I feel increasingly helpless.

Come on Henry wake up! Wake up! I pray.

"Okay, everyone. Drop six."

The sixth drop of sodium pentothal disappears into the line. Dr. Jaffe speaks to Henry in a commanding voice trying to will him awake.

"Henry, do you hear me?" He asks more forcefully.

As I watch the doctor reset the stopwatch, Henry suddenly catapults himself upright and looks at the doctors and nurses. There is a collective gasp among all of us as if we've just witnessed Lazarus rising from his grave. Dr. Jaffe, who remains stoic, speaks to Henry.

"Henry, can you hear me?" he asks gently.

Henry turns his head to focus on Dr. Jaffe, raising both arms and slamming them onto the bed.

"Of course, I can hear you. I ain't deaf!"

A wave of relief washes over me.

That's my Henry!

"Henry, do you know where you are?"

"Looks like a hospital with all of you white coats," he responds gruffly.

"Do you know what date it is?"

"How the hell should I know? There ain't no calendar here."

Henry looks perplexed and annoyed, but I can't help but smile. *Oh, yes. This is the old Henry.*

Satisfied that he's alert and oriented, Dr. Jaffe nods at me.

"Henry, do you know me?" I ask.

Henry looks at me and smiles. "Hey, Bob. What the hell am I doing here?"

"It's a long story, Henry, but we think you took a drug that has some nasty side effects. We don't know what it was. Do you know what you took?"

Henry shakes his head. "Don't remember taking anything. Think I was drinking with my son and, you know, smoking some stuff. Think we might have had a fight. It's all very fuzzy."

"You know, I'm feeling kind of tired," he says, yawning. "I'm gonna close my eyes for a while."

Henry lies back, rests his head on the pillows, and quickly falls asleep. Again, the nurse notes the time.

"It's the pentothal," says Dr. Jaffe, standing tall. "But even though we don't know what he took, it's pretty clear that this is a drug-induced delirium, and given his positive response to the pentothal, I believe we can treat it with some other medications."

I watch as the nurses remove the IV and the technicians wheel the sleeping Henry back to his room. Before I return to my office to handle another crisis admission, Dr. Jaffe pulls me aside.

"Thanks for your help, Bob. It was very useful. I will keep you posted on Henry's progress."

The staff and I have developed a working rhythm with one another, and I feel more settled in my position as the *Friday consultant*. Stepping into my early morning groove, I begin processing intake forms when Dr. Jaffe calls to inform me of Henry's status.

"Henry is doing really well," he says. "He's up, walking around and talking everyone's head off. I think he will be ready for discharge next week. Can you make the arrangements? He needs outpatient substance abuse treatment, although, with his history, I don't think he'll go."

"Let me see what I can do, and thanks for letting me see everything. The pentothal and all."

Dr. Jaffe laughs.

"Yeah. I haven't done that in a long time. It was quite the show, wasn't it? But it worked. Designer drugs! They are going to be a big problem for us. We don't know what's in them, how they work, or what their effects are, so we are not going to know how to treat them. We got lucky this time, and Henry got very, very lucky. Please tell him that for me."

"I will and, again, thanks."

"My pleasure, Bob."

The next week, Henry and I meet in my outpatient office for discharge planning. Even though he's recovered from his delirium, I want to arrange both outpatient psychotherapy and substance abuse treatment for him for one simple reason: He's leaving the safety of the hospital. After briefly discussing the treatment plan with him, we unpack the events that transpired before he arrived.

"Henry, do you remember much about what got you into the hospital?" I ask.

"Not much. It's all kind of fuzzy. Bits and pieces. Like a dream. Can't quite recall all the details."

"Do you remember calling me from the phone booth?" I ask, trying to jog his memory.

"I did?" he asks, looking puzzled. "Don't recall that at all..."

"Do you remember being in the hospital and not being able to walk?"

He fidgets in his seat uncomfortably.

"Really? I couldn't walk? No. Don't remember. I really couldn't walk. Wow."

I am not surprised that Henry is unable to recall this information since memories are stored in a chemical state in the brain before being encoded into a physical neurocircuit. If the biochemistry is disrupted either by a physical event, either traumatic or chemical, the memory is never stored and, therefore, cannot be recalled.

I decide to evaluate if he remembers when he came out of his delirium during the sodium pentothal procedure.

"Henry, do you remember when you had the IV and we talked?"

"Don't remember talking to you, but I kind of remember a bunch of white coats standing around me. Again, it's all sort of fuzzy."

He pauses and then asks, "I really couldn't walk?"

"Yep. You were crawling around and didn't know where you were."

"Wow, that's wild. I don't recall any of it. Dr. Jaffe told me I took some kind of drug, but I don't remember doing it."

"Yes, we think it was some type of special drug someone cooked up. We don't know much about it, but it can have weird effects like what happened to you. It's called a designer drug."

Henry suddenly sits upright in his chair, and his face reddens with anger.

"That son of a bitch! It was my goddamn son and his goddamn biker gang friends! They are always messing with that sort of shit. I think he wanted to fuck with me since we'd been fighting. We were drinking at the house, and we got in an argument like usual when we drink. I bet he slipped it in my cup!"

"Yes, that is exactly what I was thinking, Henry. Your son and his biker friends gave you a designer drug they cooked up."

As we both absorb the enormity of this realization, I see Henry's expression change. The anger that was there a moment ago has evolved into something more like primal desire. It's the same involuntary change I noticed in the lab with the subjects diagnosed with alcoholism.

"Designer drug. I wonder if he has any more?"

"Henry!" I shout.

Half smiling, he stands up and walks out the door.

"Be seeing you, Bob," he says, giving a half salute.

～

As Dr. Jaffe predicted, Henry never followed up with any treatment, but he also never showed up again as one of my crisis consults. The curious part of me has always wondered if he found any more designer drugs or how this event affected the relationship between him and his son.

The research I was conducting on the relapse rates among patients with substance abuse problems also found that noncompliance with treatment recommendations to be common, especially early in recovery, due to the same unconscious neuropsychological factors associated with relapse as well as the disruptive effects of the substances the patients were using. Also, the rates of noncompliance skyrocket, when, as in Henry's case, the patient's substance use is comorbid[7] with another psychiatric condition, such as post-traumatic stress.

Even though I was not surprised that Henry did not follow-up on my treatment recommendations, the feeling that I had failed to reach him triggered unsettling emotions within me—sadness for the lost opportunity to help him control his substance issues and apprehension that had it not been for Dr. Jaffe's intervention, Henry could have remained in a state for delirium for the rest of his life.

Ultimately, his noncompliance left me feeling humbled. His addiction reminded me that I was no longer in the black and white world of my government investigations but was operating in the murky environment of the human mind—a world in which treatment can be overridden by primitive and survivalist impulses to avoid pain.

---

7. Comorbid: Comorbidity is the existence of more than one disease or condition within an individual at the same time.

Questions for Consideration

1. Considering that designer drugs are made to circumvent detection and, by extension, existing laws, what regulatory strategies could be implemented to control these substances? In what ways are current policies limited in addressing these issues? How would you address it?
2. In your opinion, is relapse a personal failure due to lack of willpower, or is there evidence of a deeper neurological issue yet to be addressed?
3. From your perspective, to what extent can modern technology play a role in addiction recovery? What ethical concerns could be raised with regards to its usage?
4. In Henry's case, how do his personal relationships both prevent and enable addiction?
5. How did Henry's awareness (or lack thereof) of his own trauma affect his addiction? What challenges does a double diagnosis pose for treatment?
6. In what ways is addiction a universal human struggle (i.e., technology, sugar/junk food, escapism), and how can that inform therapeutic practices with regards to treatment?
7. Do you think that Henry ever recovered? In your opinion, should the author and the doctors have done more to help him? What do you see in Henry's case that they may have missed?
8. Do you feel that the science of the time limited Henry's recovery? After resuscitating him, was his success dependent on faith, science, or personal choice?

9. In your opinion, do you think that Henry's
   environment contributed to his success or failure in
   his treatment? What options at the time did he
   have to receive further treatment, and what options
   exist now that may have contributed to his
   recovery in a positive manner?

THE STREET PREACHER

*"The beauty of religious mania is that
it has the power to explain everything."*

— STEPHEN KING, 1978

VA Medical Center
Newington, Connecticut, 1984

THE SUN IS SHINING, and it's a beautiful, crisp spring day—the kind that makes me glad to be alive. Despite the cheerful weather, neither the mood nor the energy of the clinic reflect its splendor. It's my second year as the *Friday consultant*, and the Mental Hygiene Clinic is undergoing a significant transition with the hiring of Dr. M, a new psychiatrist to be its director. The previous one, Dr. Nelson, with whom I had an excellent working relationship, left to take a research position at the National Institute of Mental Health (NIMH).

Sitting at my desk, I reflect on my first day as the *Friday consultant*. Dr. Nelson had sensed my trepidation about the demands of the role and pulled me aside to share his wisdom.

"Look, Bob, I've known you since you were an intern, and I trust your judgment. You know how things operate here. If you need my assistance, come and get me, but if you think a patient needs to be admitted, you don't need my approval. Just call Dr. Dominick on inpatient, and he'll take care of it."

This collaborative approach stands in stark contrast to Dr. M's[1] method, which is dogmatic and imperial. A skeletally thin man of average height with thinning black hair, a mustache and a goatee; he's aloof, taciturn, and prickly. From the moment he arrived, he made it clear that he was the one in charge and that we were there to follow his orders, which are issued with an odd accent and quirky speech patterns.

Complicating matters further, he has a hostile attitude toward veterans. He doesn't trust them and has expressed his belief that they're trying to buck the system for personal gain (i.e., additional benefits and services).

Dr. M also doesn't trust the clinical staff. He thinks they are easily manipulated by veterans, particularly with respect to inpatient admissions, and continues to second-guess our decisions. He has now mandated that all inpatient admissions be approved by him, causing staff morale to plummet.

Making matters worse, he also has a strained relationship with Dr. Dominick, who he feels has been too liberal with patient admissions. The tension between these two has risen to such high levels that now, instead of making a simple phone

---

1. Name has been changed.

call to admit a patient, we have to operate like a federal bureaucracy—a memory I've tried to forget.

He is particularly suspicious of me and my role as the Friday crisis consultant and, despite repeated attempts by Dr. Daniels to explain the need for the position and its approval by chief of psychology, Dr. M. insists that there is no need for the position if we control the number of inpatients. Consequently, my interactions with Dr. M have been tense, frequently involving a grueling inquisition about each patient in need of admission.

Patient complaints have also skyrocketed, but administration appears to be either oblivious to his negative impact or actually supportive of his direct authority over all clinical activity. In a very real sense, Dr. M is a king, and we are his subjects.

With my frustration heightened over his rigid, controlling, and suspicious approach, I worry about the inpatient admissions process and the atmosphere surrounding Newington's traditionally collegial and patient-centered approach toward veterans. I rub my eyelids contemplating my future at Newington, when the clinic secretary, Helen, knocks on my office door.

Helen has been the clinic secretary since I arrived, but Dr. Daniels tells me that she's worked at the clinic before he or any of other staff started here. She's a fixture. All of the patients know Helen, and most like her. She's also pretty unshakeable, but today the usually unflappable Helen looks visibly anxious, which raises my already escalating stress levels.

"Bob, there is a patient here for admission. His name is Mike[2] and his family is with him. I have put him in the big meeting room. You'd better get in there fast before something happens. He is a bit...wild."

---

2. Name has been changed.

"A bit wild? What do you mean?" I ask.

"Just go in!" she replies, pointing toward the big room. "You'll see."

Admission evaluations are usually done either in my office or a small consulting room, but if a patient is agitated or aggressive, we use a larger meeting room, so we have space to maneuver. This reduces the risk of physical injury.

Entering the meeting room and seeing Mike for the first time, Helen's cryptic remark *You'll see* creeps into my mind as I observe the 6'3" man before me. Mike is in his late twenties and has wavy blonde hair that rests at his shoulders and a bushy beard and mustache. His eyes are a violet shade of blue and pierce with ferocity.

While his attire—a monochromatic brown leather ensemble with a broad-brimmed leather hat—is interesting, it's the Bible cradled in his right arm that's most striking. A twelve-by-eighteen-inch version, akin to a coffee table Bible, it's covered in the same brown leather as his clothes complete with identical raw hide stitching embossed in the form of a cross.

He is accompanied by his father, who stands around 5'6" and a stout young man all of 5' tall whom I presume to be his younger brother.

After observing him for a few moments as he paces around the room muttering to himself, I decide to talk to him standing up since it's unlikely he'll want to sit. His violet-blue eyes lock on to me like a hawk lasering in on its prey, and he strides over to me before I can introduce myself. His face is oddly contorted as if he is trying to contain a powerful energy inside of him that's fighting to come out. Pointing his left index finger into my face.

"I...want...to...return...my...military identity...to the president of the United States," he says in a hoarse, strained voice.

The energy within him intensifies. "And I want to do it right now!"

The mental energy and grandiosity that patients like Mike exhibit during episodes of mania can be psychologically contagious, briefly inducing fantastical and absurd thoughts and feelings in those around them. Up against Mike's towering stature, I find myself contemplating how I can grant his wish. *Can I take his ID? Can I call someone? Can I call the White House this late on a Friday?*

Thankfully, these thoughts are transient and are rapidly overridden by my perception of how emotionally distraught Mike is feeling.

"Mike, why do you want to return your ID to the president of the United States?" I ask.

He glares at me holding the Bible between us with both hands like a shield.

"Because God has told me to do it! And I must do it right now!" he shouts in a rasping, guttural tone.

The explosiveness of his energy shakes me to my core, and I sense that if I ask more questions, not only will I escalate his agitation, but I may cause him to lash out physically.

"Okay, Mike. I can see that this is important. Let me see what I can do about it."

Thinking that I might be able to diffuse the situation, I turn to his father in hopes of gathering some collateral information.

"How long has your son been like this?" I ask.

The father looks at me with tears welling up in his eyes.

"My son! My son!" he wails.

However, the next words he utters are in what I can only deduce is Polish. Mike's last name was of Polish origin, and I quickly realize that his father does not speak English fluently. With no one to translate for us, he won't be able to help.

Mike continues to pace and mumble to himself in the background. Feeling an increasing sense of desperation, I turn to his younger brother, but before I can ask him a question, he lets out a shrill, ear-splitting laugh. The psychiatric problems in this family are apparently not just limited to Mike.

Mike's voice suddenly grows louder. "I want to return my military identity to the president of the United States! Now!"

Sensing his agitation is growing, I realize that my options for dealing with this crisis are limited, and it is time for action.

Turning back to him, I say, "Okay, Mike. I am going to work on that right now, but I'll have to make a few calls first. Wait here, while I go set things up." This seems to calm him for a moment, and he nods in acknowledgement.

As I exit the meeting room, my suspicion, even from this brief interaction, is that Mike is experiencing a manic episode. However, without his clinical history, it's impossible to rule out other diagnoses such as paranoid schizophrenia or a delusional disorder[3] or whether this is a drug-induced reaction. What is clear is that he needs to be admitted to the hospital for his and others' safety, so, with a sense of impending doom knowing Dr. M's attitudes toward veterans and inpatient admissions, I dutifully head to his office.

Dr. M has his door closed, which is typical for him. After several unanswered knocks, I finally hear the word "Enter" spoken in an imperious tone—a stark contrast to the collegiate demeanor used by the other supervisors.

Expecting to have an unpleasant experience, I nervously

---

3. Delusional disorder, previously called paranoid disorder, is characterized as having one or more fixed false beliefs based on an inaccurate interpretation of an external reality despite evidence to the contrary.

open the door and enter Dr. M's domain. The window blinds are closed, and the only light emanating from the space comes from his desk lamp, causing shadows to dance across the floor and walls. He sits in the dimness behind his desk reading a medical journal. This piques my interest because, out of all the clinical directors at the hospital, he's the only one not involved in any of the research at the medical college.

"Yes, what is it, Gillespie?" he asks without looking up from the journal.

"Dr. M, there's a patient in the meeting room. He's very agitated. All I can get out of him is that he demands to return his military ID to the president. His father and younger brother are with him but can't help because the father doesn't speak English and the brother appears to have his own mental health issues. I believe the patient probably has bipolar disorder and is experiencing a manic episode although we will need a tox screen[4] to rule out drugs or alcohol. In any event, he's escalating, and he could become a danger to himself or someone else. I recommend that he be admitted promptly."

I cringe, waiting for his response.

"In my opinion," I add in the same tone I had used hundreds of times with my partner, "this guy is very close to losing it, and I am concerned that if we don't admit him now, he is going to blow up right here in the clinic. Also, he's big and I don't think he'll cooperate, so we're probably going to need a patient assistance team[5] to be able to do this safely."

---

4. Tox screen: Also known as a *drug test* or *toxicology test* analyzes blood and other bodily tissue to determine the presence of alcohol and other substances including legal and illegal.

5. A patient assistance team in this context is a rapid response team consisting of a group of designated nurses and behavioral techs who have been selected for their large size and have been trained to operate as a group to de-escalate situations without injuring the patient. The team is typically led by a physician, and in psychiatric crises, the physician is usually a psychiatrist.

Dr. M looks up from his journal and shakes his head slowly.

"Gillespie, always with the crisis! Always with the admission recommendation! No! I be deciding that," he says, his voice dripping with sarcasm. "These veterans always be trying to trick us. I no be being fooled by him, and I no be admitting him until I be talking to him and be finding out what he be trying to do. I also not be needing any assistance to do this. Be taking me now to this veteran!" He barks as he gets up from his desk.

This is not going to go well. I'm tempted to argue with him about the patient assistance team, especially with Mike's agitation rising, but every minute counts, so I decide to follow orders.

When we enter the meeting room, Dr. M sees Mike and strides over to him with authority. I place myself next to the door ready to call for help just in case the situation escalates. Without introducing himself, Dr. M presses his right index finger into Mike's chest. The noticeable height difference between them makes Mike look like a giant.

It isn't good to poke a giant.

"You be telling me what is going on," Dr. M orders with his chin in the air.

With the Bible in his hands, Mike glares at Dr. M and shoves the Bible into his face.

"I want...to return my military ID...to the president of the United States...and I want to do it now!"

"You no be talking the crazy talk to me! You be telling me the truth, or I no be talking with you!" Dr. M immediately replies punctuating each word with more finger pokes.

"I...want...to...return...my military identity to the president of the United States...and I want to do it right now!" Mike repeats, inhaling deeply between each word.

Ignoring his increasing agitation, Dr. M dismisses him with a wave of his hand and turns to his father.

"You be making the crazy talk, and I no be talking to you anymore. I now be talking to your father who be telling me what is going on."

Before I have a chance to remind Dr. M that the father doesn't understand English, he moves toward him.

"You now be telling me what is going on with your son," he says, shaking his finger in the man's face.

Mike's father clearly distressed and feeling helpless, replies, "My son! My son!" before again speaking rapidly in Polish.

Dr. M quickly cuts him off with a regal wave of his hand.

"You be speaking the English to me correctly or you no be speaking at all!"

At this point, I can feel the tension in the room increasing as Mike's father starts to cry and his little brother explodes in another bout of hysterical laughter. I notice a change in Mike's posture. His stance has become so erect that he almost seems to grow in size. He then stomps over to Dr. M who appears to shrink in both stature and ego. Leaning down, his facial muscles clench and contort with each word sounding like a punch to a jaw.

"Don't...talk...to...my...father...that...way!"

Dr. M is frozen with fear, terrified by the intensity of Mike's manic energy. Towering over him with the coffee-table size Bible still under his right arm, Mike leans down and grabs Dr. M by his white lab coat and lifts him off the ground so that his feet dangle in the air.

"I told you! I want to return my military identity to the president of the United States, and I want to do it now!"

I step to the open door of the meeting room and yell to Helen.

"Call for the patient assistance team. STAT![6] Dr. M is in trouble!"

Helen pushes a few buttons on her telephone console and speaks into the receiver. I hear her voice broadcast over the hospital's loudspeaker system.

"Patient assistance team to the main conference room, Mental Hygiene Clinic. STAT!"

Stepping back into the meeting room, I approach Mike, staying out of arms reach.

"Mike! Release Dr. M!" I say in a loud, authoritative voice, which has no effect on him at all as he begins to shake Dr. M repeatedly.

"I want to return my military identity to the president of the United States now!"

Within three minutes of Helen's call, six large men alongside Dr. Dominick march into the clinic. I quickly explain to them that the patient is having a manic episode and has physically assaulted Dr. M. They nod and enter the room without a word.

The team maintains a careful distance from Mike as they position themselves for the take down. When Mike sees them coming, he drops Dr. M to the floor and raises his Bible in front of him like a shield. Shaken, Dr. M retreats to a corner of the meeting room where Mike's father and brother are watching in horror. I quickly run to him to make sure that he's uninjured.

As the team now tightens the circle around Mike, one of them deploys a piece of equipment that I have only seen at the VA—an alternative to the classic straight jacket—a canvas sleeping bag.

---

6. "Stat" is a medical term indicating that the urgency of a task or a situation requires swift action and is derived from the Latin word "statim," which means "instantly" or "immediately."

Intimidated by the show of force[7], Mike stands motionless repeating his demands about his military ID.

As they move within reach of Mike, he starts to back up. Then, one of the team members signals, and they swiftly grab Mike's arms and his legs while another member prepares the canvas bag on the floor. The tussle causes Mike to drop his Bible, which Dr. Dominick picks up and respectfully places on a table. With Mike safely immobilized, the other four team members place him on top of the canvass as the fifth team member holds his head, so he doesn't bang it on the ground. Mike continues to struggle and shout.

"I want to return my military identity to the president of the United States!"

Carrying a syringe of Haldol, Dr. Dominick approaches Mike as the team restrains his arms and legs. He injects the medicine into him intramuscularly[8] while Mike thrashes against the patient assistance team. The medicine would calm most patients instantly, but, to our horror, it has no effect on Mike. Everyone is now a bit nervous.

Ready for battle, Dr. Dominick reloads the syringe and administers another dose.

"One more time!" he shouts.

The second dose doesn't work either, but a third has the desired effect. Mike's body relaxes even though his eyes continue to dart around the room—an indicator that he's still highly alert despite the medication.

In a well-rehearsed choreography, the crisis response team zips the canvas bag over Mike while a tech brings a gurney. They gently lift him and begin to wheel him down the corridor

---

7. Show of force: A demonstration of power intended to warn or intimidate an opponent by displaying a great number of people or resources.
8. Intramuscularly: Within a muscle. In an intramuscular injection, the needle is passed deeply into a muscle before the fluid is injected.

toward the elevator. With his arm wrapped around Dr. M, Dr. Dominick escorts him back to his office for a debrief.

"Bob, call the unit and let them know what is coming their way," he says as he walks toward the door. "Tell them to keep him restrained until I get there to sort things out. Also, try to get his father and brother to understand what's going on."

Feeling a sense of relief that the circus is over, I pick up the phone to call the charge nurse on the psychiatric unit.

Suddenly, I see Astrid arriving at the clinic out of the corner of my eye. She's here for our weekly post-clinic date night. I nod hello to her while holding the phone to my ear, but as she smiles back, the six members of the patient assistance team suddenly come sprinting down the hallway nearly knocking her over. To my shock, a grisly scene right out of the 1930s *Mummy* movie unfolds before me. Behind the terrified patient assistant team is Mike, who is loping awkwardly with the canvas bag wrapped around his left foot[9] bellowing incoherently.

Seeing Astrid's eyes widen in horror, I quickly yank her[10] away from the drama and shove her into my office. Then, squeezing the emergency phone tightly with both hands, I shout at the charge nurse on the psychiatric unit.

"Send another patient assistance team! STAT!"

Twelve men and Dr. Dominick now surround Mike in the hallway. He continues to fight, but they are able to successfully restrain him, put him back in a working canvas bag, and lift him onto the gurney. As they whisk him down the corridor, I

---

9. I was later told that there was a defect in the canvass bag's straps and when they tried to maneuver the gurney on to the elevator in a rage, he had burst free.
10. Astrid later asked rather quizzically at dinner, "Does this kind of thing go on often?" I don't recall my reply to her, but I'm sure I must have been thinking *Just another day as the Friday consultant!*

speak in a combination of broken English and unofficial sign language to Mike's father in an attempt reassure him that his son will be well cared for. I'm not sure how much he understands but based on his nodding and the look of relief on his face, I think he gets the idea. The little brother, not so much.

I never saw Dr. M again after the incident. He remained secluded in his office for the rest of the day, and when I returned the following Friday, he was gone. Officially, there was never any explanation as to why he left, but there was a rumor that, after an extended leave, he had been transferred to another VA hospital in a nonclinical role. Dr. Dominick's senior resident was temporarily assigned to be the medical director of the outpatient clinic, which made patient admissions a lot easier.

I visited Mike each week while he was an inpatient and at the end of his second week met with Dr. Dominick in his office to assess Mike's progress.

Sitting behind a desk cluttered with patient files, Dom leans back with his hands behind his head and gives me his assessment.

"Bob, his tox screens were all negative, so I am inclined to agree with your diagnosis of a manic episode secondary to bipolar disorder. I've started him on an initial medication regime of antipsychotic medications and lithium. As his mania and delusional thinking begin to recede, I'll slowly titrate[11] and eliminate the antipsychotic medication and place him on a maintenance dose of lithium for long-term treatment. Already,

____

11. Titration of a medicine means to slowly increase or decrease the dose by very small amounts over time.

he is a far cry from the man who needed three powerful injections of Haldol to subdue him."

Under Dr. Dominick's treatment, Mike's condition continued to improve, and at the end of six weeks he was ready to be discharged. When I meet with him in my office to plan his outpatient treatment, I notice a dramatic change in his demeanor from how he presented during my intake. Dressed in jeans, a paisley shirt, and boots, the leather clothes and huge embossed Bible are gone. Thankfully, the manic energy he came in with is no longer present either, and he's able to calmly explain what happened to him.

Mike begins by sharing about his relationship with his father who had emigrated from Poland in the early 1950s to flee from the communists.

"My father whose name is Michal or, in English, Michael, was a dentist in Poland. Never mastered English after coming to America and so he had to work at low skill jobs his whole life. I think he was always a bit depressed and withdrawn. Maybe because of that or the language barrier, I was never close to him emotionally,".

Hhen shifts to talking about his relationship with his mother.

"Shortly after emigrating, my father met and married my mother, Catherine, who was an American. Unlike with my father, I was very close to my mother. She was a devout Catholic and had made the Catholic church an important fixture for our family. We went to church together every Sunday and on all the holy days. As a child, I attended a Catholic elementary school, but when I became a teenager, I went to a public high school," he says, leaning back in his chair with a hint of sadness in his voice.

"After graduating high school, I enlisted in the Army, and when I completed basic and advanced infantry training, I was deployed to Germany. I liked the structure and discipline of the Army and, at first, things went well until at the end of my first year in Germany. I was arrested after driving a jeep recklessly around the local town near the base. When they realized I was having a psychotic episode, they took me to the hospital instead of jail, which resulted in me being diagnosed with bipolar disorder and eventually led to a medical discharge from the military. When I got home, I was also supposed to follow-up with the VA for medical care, but since I was feeling fine, I never did."

In describing the next four years, it appears that Mike experienced several hypomanic episodes[12] followed by periods of depression but never sought any treatment and did not have another full manic episode until several months before his father brought him to the clinic that Friday afternoon.

This episode appears to have been triggered by the death of his mother after a painful battle with cancer approximately six months before his visit to the VA.

"When Mom died, it was like my whole world fell apart. I felt overwhelmed with grief, and I couldn't function. Then my emotions and thinking changed. My grief suddenly faded, and I began experiencing an intense religious zeal I had never felt before. Initially, it felt fulfilling—energizing even—but eventually this initial enthusiasm morphed into a force that I could no longer control, and I started believing I was on a mission from God to save the unsaved by preaching the Bible. It felt like the 'religious epiphanies' the prophets had in all the Bible stories I'd read."

Interrupting him, I ask, "Mike can you recall what it was like for you when you experienced this change?"

---

12. Hypomanic episodes involve elation and hyperactivity that is less severe than in mania. Typically, these do not require hospitalization.

"It was like being in a dream. I couldn't get the thoughts out of my head. I was driven by them, and, for a while, I felt incredibly empowered. Slowly, though, even these the feelings changed, and I became consumed with the idea that I had been specially chosen, like an Old Testament prophet. Then, one day, I saw a drawing of a prophet in a book. He was dressed in leather holding a huge Bible with a cross on it, and I knew that this was who I had been chosen to be. I began dressing up in leather and spent hours sewing a cover embossed with a cross on a large Bible I had purchased. I quit my job doing carpentry and began preaching in the streets and in local seedy bars in downtown Hartford because that was where the sinners were.

"It was in the bars that the trouble began. In the streets, most people just generally avoided me, but in the bars, it was a different story. The patrons didn't welcome my fire-and-brimstone exhortations and so I got into a few fights. It was after I got thrown out of a bar one night after a particularly bad fight that I experienced what felt like a revelation. The reason I could not save the unsaved was because *I* had not yet been purified. I was still a sinner because I was in the Army, and that identity was incompatible with doing the divine work I had been chosen for. It was all I could think of. It became all mixed up in my head with saving the unsaved and being chosen. I started to feel a compelling need to act because if I didn't, I would be damned for all eternity. The only action that could save me was to renounce my military identity directly to the person in charge—the Commander in Chief, the president of the United States himself—but I didn't know how to go about doing it."

According to Mike, coming to the VA was his father's idea.

"I think my father was alarmed at my preaching work, especially after I kept getting beaten up. He convinced me that since I was a veteran and the VA was part of the government, that maybe you guys could help me return my military identity. It made sense to me somehow, and I decided to come here. What happened after I arrived is a bit fuzzy, but I do recall talking with you and that other doctor."

He pauses, as if searching his memory for the forgotten details.

"I have talked to Dr. Dominick and my father about what happened, and they have filled in most of the details for me, but it still feels like a dream. I feel really bad about what I did to that other doctor. That's not like me at all. In fact, the whole thing doesn't feel like me, even though I know I did all those things. I'm feeling a lot better now, though. I'm not having any of those thoughts anymore, and I don't feel that weird energy. I think the medicine Dr. Dominick is giving me is helping a lot."

Understanding the dynamics of Mike's manic episode, I decide to shift the focus of our conversation to his outpatient treatment plan.

"Mike, the condition you have can create episodes like you just had, but it can be treated with a combination of medication and psychotherapy so that they don't happen again. The medicine keeps things stable, and the therapy is like an educational course that helps you come to understand how your version of the condition works so you can eventually learn to manage it yourself."

Mike nods at the arrangement.

Observing the man before me, I am struck by the lucidity of our conversation. The mania I witnessed that day in the meeting room has completely disappeared. The man who held Dr. M in the air with nothing more than sheer physical willpower is now calm, coherent, and self-aware. For me, this has always been both the most remarkable and the most troubling aspect of bipolar disorder.

At present, we do not have a clear understanding of the causes of bipolar disorder. Like schizophrenia, there is significant evidence from family and twin studies that it has a genetic component. It also appears to follow the diathesis-stress model[13], which is a genetic predisposition that's triggered by environmental factors such as stress or trauma.

In Mike's case, it appears that the event that caused his manic episode was the death of his mother. A devoutly religious woman who instilled her values into him combined with the grief he experienced over her loss triggered his underlying vulnerability, which manifested into a religious transformation. This created an intense emotional conflict within him when he perceived that his military experience was at odds with his newfound spiritual identity.

While identifying these triggers can help patients make sense of their specific episodes, it is not necessary for treating the disorder. The most effective treatment of a bipolar episode is not a matter of discovering a deep, dark secret or uncovering repressed memories (also known as Freudian catharsis[14]) but rather recognizing the symptoms indicating the onset of a manic or depressive episode, properly managing medication

---

13. The *diathesis-stress model* is a theory that explains the development of certain specific mental disorders as a result of the interaction between a predispositional, generally genetic, vulnerably (diathesis) that creates an inherent susceptibility to the emergence of the disorder in response to environmental stressors. Environmental stressors can include transitional life stressors such as puberty, leaving home, giving birth, interpersonal loss, and psychological trauma, or physical stressors such as serious illness or pain.

14. In psychology catharsis refers to releasing or expressing repressed emotions or feelings. It was first introduced by Freud and his early partner, Josef Breuer in 1895 in their book *Studies on Hysteria*. They defined it as "the process of reducing or eliminating a complex by recalling it to conscious awareness and allowing it to be expressed."

intake, and providing emotional support during and after the episode. In helping the patient learn to self-regulate, this approach is similar to the treatment of other chronic illnesses like diabetes.

To facilitate this process, patients, doctors, and therapists usually work through several manic-depressive cycles before there's enough information to manage them adequately. This usually involves a trial-and-error process of testing the medications and dosages before the patient and their physician know what works best, as each individual responds to medication differently, and the severity of the disorder can vary from person to person. The primary role of psychotherapy in this process is to help the patient cope with the destructive effects of their manic-depressive cycles as well as the stresses of everyday life.

Mike's case also presented a different type of difficulty for me as a clinician—that of differentiating a true religious experience from a manic episode.

The history of religion is replete with stories of people being talked to by God. In the Judeo-Christian tradition, such descriptions date back to Abraham and Moses. While these days I use the lens of science, and particularly neuroscience, as a means of explaining my own experiences, I recognize that understanding such spiritual experiences may be beyond the scope of this method, as they are not easily subjectable to scientific analysis.

Further, to broadly attach pejorative labels, such as mania, to such historical descriptions or to all episodes of religious awakenings or religious ecstasy, some of which can be quite beneficial to an individual, is a counterproductive act of clinical hubris. Yet, being able to differentiate a true religious experience from mania is important given how dangerous manic episodes can be to the patient and those around them.

There is no perfect way to resolve this dilemma. It is, however, important to establish a therapeutic alliance and to be respectful and sensitive to a patient's religious beliefs. This allows for an exploratory process to unfold where they can examine the context of how these beliefs developed and are currently being manifested. This can give clues as to whether the patient is experiencing mania or something else. In Mike's case that's consistent with the diathesis-stress model, his was mania and the timing of his religious experience were connected to the death of his mother.

Further, in speaking with individuals who claim to have experienced religious transformations rather than manic episodes, I've noticed that the identity transformation tends to endure over time and feels consistent with who they are. In contrast, the identity crisis Mike experienced dissipated once he was stabilized with a combination of medication and therapy. His messianic thoughts vanished and, while he still remained a devout Catholic, he recognized that those thoughts were the *not me* version of him, and he felt disturbed at having had them.

Other clues that support mania as opposed to a religious awakening are his unusual manner of dressing, the recklessness of his actions, and the absurdity of his request regarding his military ID. All of these suggest the presence of disorganized and erratic thinking, which is not typical of a true religious experience as they've been described to me. To the contrary, individuals who have had religious awakenings report that their thinking becomes "reorganized" by the experience.

There was also the feeling of emotional explosiveness during Mike's episode. This is a palpable energy that one can feel when interacting with a patient having a manic episode, and, based on my experience, this is not common with religious awakenings. Manic energy is big energy, and when I'm in the room with a patient like Mike who is experiencing mania, regardless of the content of their thinking, it's their energy that I can feel. I can only describe it as a physical force emanating from them that is both undeniable and overwhelming. It's like being in a room with an angry, unpredictable giant, and once a person has experienced it, they never forget it.

On a deeper level, however, I understand the seductive power of the religious experience that Mike had. Like him, I was raised in the Catholic faith and attended a Catholic elementary school where the nuns told me the stories of biblical figures and saints being spoken to by God. I can distinctly remember as a child not only being enchanted by such tales but also being envious since I had not had such an experience and really wanted to. While I've learned to acquire my insights in a more controlled and measured manner, I'm not completely immune to the allure of the possibility of such experiences.

Questions for Consideration

1. Considering Dr. M's personal biases toward veterans, do you believe he should have been retrained or removed from his role as clinical supervisor? When does personal bias cross the line in a professional setting?
2. In what way did the hierarchal structure of the hospital and potential fear of retaliation preserve the status quo and prevent the author from confronting discriminatory practices?
3. The author mentions that Dr. M could have received support from his superiors for his

regimented and strict policies on patient admissions. In what ways can aspiring professionals develop the courage and skill to confront unethical practices?

4. What do you feel was the primary driver of Mike's miraculous recovery—ongoing treatment or medication? In your opinion, would Mike eventually be able to ween himself off of either?

5. Do you think that Mike would stop taking his medication to experience mania again?

6. Are spiritual experiences often misdiagnosed as mania, or is mania misinterpreted as a spiritual revelation? In what ways do you think the author's culture and upbringing shaped his opinion around this experience?

7. Do you think that mania is the brain's way of reaching for an experience beyond ordinary human awareness?

8. What aspects of bipolar disorder were so troubling to the author and why?

THE FOURTH WALL

"...I love you - love you as I have never loved any living thing. From the moment I met you I loved you, loved you blindly, adoringly, madly! You didn't know it then - you know it now."

— OSCAR WILDE, 1911

WEST HARTFORD, Connecticut, 1984

It is the night of my first son's christening, and the festivities are in full swing. Family, friends, and coworkers have all gathered together at our home in West Hartford to celebrate. However, above the melodious rhythm of music, conversation, and laughter, I start to notice a discordant noise that clashes with the mood of the party and leaves me with a sense of unease. The sound is unrelenting and disturbing, but no one else seems to notice.

The most influential person in my life has been my wife, Astrid, whose love, ferocious intellect, and sense of adventure has been one of the most powerful driving forces behind my career as a psychotherapist. From the moment I saw her when she was a young program director for the agency fresh out of Columbia University destined to become a most accomplished lawyer, I was completely enchanted by her—a captivation that became not just an amorous pursuit but a budding partnership.

When we met, Astrid was still toying with the idea of pursuing a part-time career in theater in New York City. As an undergraduate at Columbia University, she'd immersed herself in the performing arts and even directed a version of the medieval morality play *Every Man* for the Glastonbury Festival in England. Sensing my monkish upbringing and education, I think she took a bit of pleasure in introducing me to the theatrical arts.

I grew up on Long Island in a small town called Queens Village. My childhood community was made up primarily of working-class Irish Catholics, and almost all social activities were centered around the local church. I was educated by a group of semi-cloistered nuns in elementary school and in an all-male high school and college run by two different orders of celibate Catholic brothers. Despite its proximity to New York City, it was a sheltered, protected world—an isolated island far from the culturally rich megalopolis of the Big Apple.

In my world, live theatre didn't exist, except as silly—and often embarrassing—school plays, which were to be avoided at all costs. The only understanding of theater I had was going to the movies with my friends. It was just another form of entertainment that I never gave much thought to, but with Astrid, all that changed.

Discussing theatre with her was like taking a mind-expanding drug and entering a world that I never knew existed. As she described it, theater was not an event that was meant to be passively witnessed but an exhaustively planned and choreographed process in which every detail was meticulously calibrated for impact on the audience. One aspect in particular that piqued my curiosity was the theatrical concept of the *fourth wall.*

The fourth wall refers to an imaginary boundary during a performance that separates the audience from the actors. Since a theater stage is made up of three solid walls, the fourth wall is invisible. The actors are on one side of it interacting with each other and creating a universe that the audience observes but can never enter. Psychologically, this helps the audience suspend their disbelief for the duration of the play so that the performance has its desired effect.

Sometimes, however, the play will call for an actor to violate the fourth wall and speak directly to the audience, which, if done well, can have a powerful effect and draw them into the drama. Examples of this theatrical device are Thornton Wilder's use of the stage manager in his play, *Our Town.* Instead of only having the characters act out the story, the people living in Grover's Corner reveal the elements of the setting, and the stage manager, who is not one of the characters, moves around the stage providing exposition about the performance directly to the audience. More recently, the TV series *House of Cards* uses this technique when the main character, Frank Underwood, frequently turns to the camera, sometimes breaking from the scene in mid dialogue, to tell the viewers what he's thinking or planning.

What intrigued me about this concept was its similarity to

maintaining appropriate boundaries in psychotherapy—an issue that every new clinician receives ethical training on because of the intimacy of the therapeutic experience[1]. However, one of the boundaries in treatment that's rarely talked about is the setting. This space, usually an office or meeting room, is actually a part of the treatment. Just as in theatre, it provides an invisible boundary—a fourth wall—that's crucial for the process to be effective.

In the theatre, when the fourth wall is violated, it's usually a planned strategy designed to enhance the story. However, in psychotherapy, it's a destructive and often dangerous path that can ruin lives.

~

VA Medical Center
Newington, Connecticut, 1983

The July heat this Friday afternoon nearly takes my breath away, but even the humidity is no match for the dramatic increase in the volume of outpatients we have. Swamped, Dr. Daniels calls me into his office to ask that I take on another case.

While my primary role as the *Friday consultant* is to do diagnostic assessments for crisis admissions, we agree that, under Dr. Daniels's supervision, I can continue psychotherapy with a few patients from my internship and work as a co-therapist with him in a post-traumatic stress disorder group on Tuesday nights. Occasionally, I perform other limited clinical services, such as neuropsychological evaluations, but it's not the norm for me to assume additional caseloads for the clinic.

---

1. For example, not dating or having sex with a patient.

His request comes during a time of intense professional and personal activity. I'm working with the research team writing journal articles on our relapse research and am preparing to defend my dissertation at my university in New York. Also, Astrid and I are joyously expecting our first child, and in preparation for his arrival, we recently purchased our first home in West Hartford. To help finance this, I'm working a second job outside of the VA directing a psychiatric shelter[2] for chronically mentally ill patients at a local community mental health center in the neighboring town of New Britain, Connecticut.

I recognize that Dr. Daniels is asking for a favor. We are both feeling the pinch, and I know he wouldn't have asked if he felt that there were any other options. I also feel compelled to do it because this is my last year as the *Friday consultant*. Dr. Daniels' guidance and kindness over the past four years have been invaluable, and this is my way of giving back.

The patient is a married female veteran in her mid-thirties named Lilly[3]. She stands about 5'4" tall and is of average weight with dark mid-length hair and brown eyes that are reminiscent of her Mexican American heritage. She has also just moved to Connecticut from Texas with her husband and was treated by the VA Medical Center in Waco. Dr. Daniels describes her as a woman suffering from recurrent severe episodes of depression with suicidal ideation but without any suicide attempts. Her medications will be managed by Dr. Dominick's chief resident, who is temporarily directing our

---

2. This was a program run by the local community mental health agency in New Britain, Connecticut. Known as The Psychiatric Shelter Program, it was designed to deal with the homelessness problem created by deinstitutionalization by providing temporary housing for recently discharged state hospital patients with chronic mental illness.
3. Name has been changed.

clinic since Dr. M's departure. My role is to provide short-term psychotherapy for her depressive episodes.

Based on her clinical records, Lilly grew up in Waco, Texas and was the youngest of six children. Her father was a career sergeant in the Army, and after high school, she followed her father's footsteps and enlisted. During her deployment in Germany, she experienced her first severe depressive episode and was hospitalized. Shortly after, she was medically discharged and returned to her home in Texas.

Unfortunately, Lilly's depressive episodes didn't stop after she returned home. She was hospitalized several times at the VA in Waco, Texas and received extensive outpatient treatment, which included a partial hospital program[4], medication, and regular psychotherapy sessions from a psychiatric resident at Baylor University.

I also learned from her records that she has been married for about five years and does not have any children. She met her husband Charles[5], who was an electrical engineer for a national firm, when she returned to Texas after her discharge from the military. Their move from Texas to Connecticut was due to his work.

Upon meeting Lilly, I have the feeling that there is something amiss with her. The emotions she exhibits during our treatment session are not congruent with her diagnosis of depression. While my primitive brain doesn't sense any imminent danger, my intuition tells me that there's more to Lilly than I can discern from her medical records.

Depressive patients in treatment usually present as

---

4. A Partial Hospital Program (PHP) is a structured outpatient treatment option for individuals with mental health or substance use disorders that provides intensive therapeutic services while allowing patients to return home at the end of the day.
5. Name has been changed.

emotionally constricted and subdued. It is generally difficult for them to talk about their thoughts and feelings, especially early in treatment, but this is not the case with Lilly. During our first session, she oscillates between feeling depressed and withdrawn to lashing out in full-blown anger and rage. She describes the Army, the VA, and, especially, her husband as aloof and uncaring. She is particularly upset with him about his job transfer that uprooted her from her family in Texas, and she is also adamant that he is not meeting her needs emotionally or sexually and is quite frank about the latter.

It's not just these emotional outbursts that sound my alarms regarding Lilly's condition. She brings into the treatment room an emotion that I cannot identify—one that's deeper and more disturbed.

After the first session with Lilly, I discuss my concerns with Dr. Daniels in clinical supervision.

"Dan, I can't quite explain it. There is a subtle disconnection between what she is saying and her emotional expression that suggests the presence of repressed thoughts and feelings. It's not *what* she's saying that's disturbing to me; it's what she isn't."

"Bob, it sounds to me like your unconscious is recognizing something in the treatment that your conscious mind hasn't yet figured out. I would keep exploring it with her. I suspect that your speculations will become clearer as her treatment progresses and the repressed material emerges," he says, reminding me to stay focused on the process.

When a patient undergoes psychotherapy, I typically ask them how they feel about the approaches and techniques they've tried in the past. In Lilly's case, she is quite clear that the treatment she received at the Waco VA has been dissatisfying and disappointing.

"I didn't like it there. When I was an inpatient, the nurses were mean to me, and I felt like a prisoner. It was a huge hospital and the whole atmosphere wasn't friendly, not like it is here. There, I felt like I was back in the Army—just a number, you know? But when I come here for treatment, everybody knows who I am. It feels like a big family, and I like you as my therapist."

Score one for us!

Lilly is particularly venomous in describing her outpatient psychotherapy with the psychiatric resident assigned to her at Waco.

"That guy is a total dud. Session after session, he just sat there and nodded. He didn't say anything! He was just like my husband—aloof, emotionally distant, and non-communicating. I wanted someone to talk with me about what I was feeling. Not just someone who sat there! Anyway, that's why I just stopped going. I was so frustrated!"

Unfortunately, this story isn't new. Patient frustration caused by "therapeutic silence" is fairly common. This is a practice that resulted from a misunderstanding of Freud's technique of free association[6] within his psychoanalytic method. Working in the Victorian culture of late 19th and early 20th century Germany, Freud struggled with the highly restrictive social conventions that prohibited people from talking

---

6. Free association is a psychoanalytic technique used to explore the unconscious mind where individuals express their thoughts, feelings, and memories without censorship or judgment. It aims to reveal hidden or repressed thoughts and emotions that may be influencing a person's behavior or causing psychological distress. The therapist listens focused on the client's words, emotional tone, body language, and patterns of speech and occasionally make interpretations.

freely about their thoughts and emotions, especially ones concerning sexuality or aggression. To counter this, he initially experimented with hypnosis but abandoned this technique because he believed it was too unreliable. He eventually chose to encourage his patients to verbalize their thoughts and feelings without self-censoring. He would sit outside of their field of vision and listen quietly so as not to distract them, and the patients would gradually reveal their deepest thoughts, memories, and feelings without fear of social ostracization or retribution.

While this may have been a useful strategy in that era, it is not as effective today because patients are usually more open and accepting of such ideas and feelings. As a result, therapeutic silence has dropped out of general clinical use, but occasionally, there will be a novice psychotherapist using it because they feel the need to emulate what they perceive as the "classic model."

Feeling confident that I will not make the same mistake[7] with Lilly, I listen as she gleefully recounts the bizarre manner in which she handled her frustration with the resident just before dropping out of treatment.

"After months of this guy nodding and not saying much, I decided it was time to get his attention. Instead of going to my scheduled appointment, I went to the fountain that was in front of the building just below his office. He had a window facing it. It was a warm summer afternoon. Jumping into the fountain, I stripped off all my clothes and began yelling his name as loud as I could saying he wasn't very good at his job. I

---

7. For me, psychotherapy is an interactive, educative, and communicative process during which both parties learn something about themselves and each other. The therapist takes an active role and doesn't just sit in a dark corner taking notes repetitiously asking, *"And how does that make you feel?"*

also said a lot of other not so complimentary things about my treatment at the Waco VA."

Momentarily stunned, I ask, "You did what?"

"Yep. Stripped naked and called out his name," she says with a smirking and flirtatious gaze in her eyes.

I begin to reconsider my criticism of the previous resident's therapeutic approach.

"Then what happened?" I ask.

"Well, eventually, the security guards came and got me out of the fountain. They took me to the ER, but by then, I had calmed down, so they didn't put me in the hospital. They released me a few hours later when my husband came to get me. He was pretty upset with me, but I didn't care. I had made my point. I never saw that resident again and never went back to psychotherapy there. We moved here shortly after and I began seeing you."

Lilly's words send shivers down my spine. My internal alert system is firing on all cylinders. Something is definitely off with Lilly, but I still don't know what to make of it. The only thing I know is that I'm not going to make the same mistake that the inexperienced psychiatric resident did. I've had a lot more training, and I can certainly manage her treatment so that she won't need to strip or jump into our fountain.

Imbued with confidence, I commence her treatment on what I perceive to be the core issue driving her depressive episodes—her dysfunctional marriage.

"Lilly, I think that right now the conflict you are having with Charles is contributing to your depression. I would like to work on improving the communication between you two. Also, I believe it will be helpful to get Charles to come so we can get his input. What do you think?"

Lilly's eyes darken. "I don't want him involved. His coming can't help you and me, Doctor."

It's early in treatment She'll come around.

She is simply trying to assert control of the process, which isn't unusual as patients are not passive participants in their own therapy. They initiate coming to see a therapist, and, even if they are confused about their symptoms, they generally have some ideas about what's causing them. Also, because patients are invited to explore their thoughts and feelings by revisiting painful memories and questioning long-standing beliefs, they can feel overwhelmed and attempt to avoid or control the process. Descriptions of this phenomena date back to Freud who coined the term *resistance*[8] in his early work on the treatment of hysteria in collaboration with Josef Breuer around 1895[9].

Over the course of our therapy sessions, Lilly's depressive symptoms appear to decrease, and her emotional expression becomes less negative. She isn't as angry and rageful as before although she remains rather hostile toward her marriage. Overall, her attitude toward life is optimistic—almost euphoric, so I am feeling good about the progress we've made.

But as they say, *pride always cometh before the fall.*

West Hartford, Connecticut, 1983

The gentle splash of the sun's early morning rays pours

---

8. Resistance refers to the phenomenon in psychotherapy where a patient consciously or unconsciously avoids discussing certain thoughts, feelings, or memories during therapy. This behavior is seen as a defense mechanism that protects the individual from confronting painful or distressing issues.

9. Freud's first use of the term *resistance* was in his book, *Studies on Hysteria* (Standard Edition, II, at pp. 278-87) which he published with Josef Breuer in 1895.

through the windows of our rental house. It's a beautiful Saturday in late autumn, and the deep greens of summer have exploded into a mosaic of red, yellow, and golden-brown colors just in time to accentuate the aroma of the wood fires. This fall is particularly magical because Astrid is in her second trimester, and we are in the process of moving into the new home in West Hartford. I'm filled with a joyous sense of new beginnings. That is, until I open the front door.

Struggling with an armful of cardboard boxes, I look up and see a small red car parked in front of our driveway. This is unusual since the rental house is at the end of a cul-de-sac, and normally no one parks here. Curious, I set the boxes on the pavement and walk toward the vehicle, thinking that they are lost and I may be able to help.

My good Samaritan thoughts quickly vanish when I see Lilly sitting in the driver's seat. I feel disoriented and confused at seeing her outside of the hospital. *This has to be some kind of mistake.*

"Lilly, what are you doing here?" I ask, immediately assuming the role of her doctor.

"I followed you home last night after our session," she replies, smiling just a little too brightly for my comfort.

"You've been here all night?" I ask in disbelief.

"Yes! I've been waiting for you!"

I feel the hackles rising on my back as adrenaline rushes through my body. I try to suppress my brain's paleomammalian response. *This is some type of cry for help. I can manage this the same as I would in a clinical setting.*

"Why did you do this, Lilly?"

Her face transforms into a maniacal grin.

"You know why. We are supposed to be together."

With my heart pounding hard in my chest, I back away from her car.

"You can't be doing this. I will only see you in the office and nowhere else," I admonish. "Do you understand?"

"Yes, of course, but we're still supposed to be together!" she says, still grinning.

"Only in the office, Lilly!" I yell, feeling her eyes, bright and intense, still fixated on me.

As I enter the house, Astrid comes to the door having witnessed the exchange between me and Lilly.

"Who was that?"

"It was one of my patients. She apparently followed me home last night after our session."

"She was outside all night in her car?" she asks with an edge of alarm.

"She's just confused about the boundaries in therapy. I've straightened her out about it. I don't think it will happen again."

"It better not. We've got a baby coming!" The alarm in her voice is replaced with an icy assertiveness.

"I know. I'll take care of it."

Nothing in my training or experience has prepared me for a patient coming to see me outside of a clinical setting, especially not at my home. What I do not fully recognize as I attempt to reassure Astrid is that the fourth wall of my clinical office no longer exists. Rather than being Lilly's therapist, I'm now an unwitting participant in an unfolding drama–one in which I'm the leading man to her leading lady.

On Monday morning, I set up a supervision session with Dr. Daniels.

"Dan, I think I can manage this and continue her treatment. She's just confused about the boundaries, but I will reinforce their importance in our next treatment session and tell her that I will only see her in the office."

Dr. Daniels no longer looks at me as a fellow psychotherapist. He has fully assumed the role of clinical supervisor.

"Bob, you cannot continue treating her," he says firmly. "I don't think you fully understand what's going on here. You're thinking she is your patient and that you are her therapist, but she doesn't think about you that way. She thinks you're her boyfriend and has some crazy idea that you're destined to be together, like some star-crossed lovers. Worse, she's not just thinking and feeling these things, which can sometimes happen in therapy; she's *acting* on them."

"But Dan, I'm her psychotherapist," I counter, still in denial.

"For God's sake, Bob. Wake up!" he interrupts, exasperated by my insistence. "In her mind, you're no longer her therapist. She followed you home, which is creepy to say the least. What's next? This type of boundary violation can be dangerous. There are instances where patients have actually killed their therapists. Doing therapy under these circumstances is not possible. So, for her sake and yours, I will arrange to have the case transferred to someone else, and I will watch this situation closely. In any event, you are not to see her again. Do you understand?"

I'm sure he is just being melodramatic.

With reluctance, I accept his decision feeling like a teenager who just received after-school detention.

Astrid and I are ecstatic to have finally moved into our new home and are relaxing together on the living room couch enjoying one of the last quiet evenings before the birth of our son. Dr. Daniels, as promised, has taken care of Lilly's transfer to another therapist and it's been a month since I've seen her. I'm feeling good that the Lilly situation is behind us.

As Astrid and I are giving each other a warm, pre-baby bliss smile, the phone rings. Grabbing the receiver with one hand, I cuddle her in my other arm and wink at her before picking up the phone.

"Hello?"

Silence. I pull the phone away from my ear to make sure it's working properly when I hear a plaintive voice whimpering.

"Why are you doing this to me?"

My heart instantly drops to the floor. *Oh my god! It's Lilly. How did she get the phone number for our new home? Does she know where we live?*

"You are supposed to be with me. You are my man, not hers. I love you."

Lilly's voice now escalates from sadness to fury.

"That bitch doesn't deserve you! She doesn't love you. You need to be with me. We are supposed to be together!"

Trying to hide my trepidation from Astrid, I remember Dr. Daniels' statement about the danger Lilly presented for me and my family.

Seething with rage, my blood begins to boil.

"Never call me again! You are no longer in treatment with me. There is no reason for any more contact. More importantly, and I need you to hear this clearly, we are not involved in a relationship! Don't call again!" I scream as I slam the phone onto the receiver.

Astrid, startled by the intensity of my reaction, gives me a questioning look.

"Who was that?"

"It was Lilly," I say, cutting straight to the point.

"What does she want?" she says, responding with an edge of anger in her tone.

Knowing that my wife is an exceptional lie detector, I explain what Lilly said, and her reaction is as predicted. She's furious, and an unspoken tension lingers between us.

As we sit in silence, the phone rings again. This time, I don't hear a distraught or angry voice on the line, only an eerie and ominous silence.

"Stop calling!" I yell, my voice filled with a combination of guilt, anger, and helplessness. No sooner than I hang up the phone, it rings again. This time Astrid answers, the fury in her voice sending shivers down my spine.

"You had better stop this now! Do not call us! Ever again!"

The calls continue for hours, so we decide to leave the phone off the hook. Lying in bed later that night exhausted, we discuss what's happening with Lilly.

"Honey, I never had to deal with anything like this with a patient. I had to deal with angry patients sure and even agitated patients. You remember the incident with Mike. But nothing like this, like being stalked."

"Yes, I know. She sounds very deluded. I'm just angry that she disturbed us at home, and on one of our last nights before the baby."

The tension between us gradually fades as both of us realize that we are now dealing with a disturbed individual. When faced with a crisis, we unite as a couple.

"So, what are you going to do about it?" Astrid asks.

"I'm not exactly sure, but I will be talking about how to handle this with Dr. Daniels tomorrow."

I call Dr. Daniels the next morning, but he shares even more frightening news.

"Bob, Lilly is definitely in the wind. She hasn't started treatment with the new psychologist either. In fact, since your last therapy session, she hasn't been to the clinic at all. Every attempt to contact her has failed. Phone calls, visitations, everything. Even the mailed notices have been returned."

The next night, the silent hang up calls begin again. Lilly either hangs up or lingers on the line for a minute or two. Also, her calls start coming later and later at night around midnight or one or two in the morning. This continues until we finally obtain an unlisted number, which curbs the harassment but makes it more difficult for friends and family to reach us.

Thankfully, though, after a few nights without harassing calls, Astrid feels more confident leaving the house for the first time. However, when she steps outside to grab the mail, she notices that there's an odd envelope addressed to her on our welcome mat. Without a stamp or return address, we're both left with an unsettling feeling. *Lilly knows where we live.*

Furious, Astrid hands the letter to me. It's a long and rambling handwritten note filled with hateful profanity against Astrid.

You are a bitch because you are preventing us from being together! You should let him go because we were destined to be together. He is my man, not yours! If you don't recognize this, you are a fucking bitch and whore!

"If I didn't know it before, I do now. She's just crazy," Astrid says, shifting into attorney mode. "With no direct threats in either the letter or the phone calls and not knowing her whereabouts, we're not going to be able to get a restraining order."

"We need to get a security system for the house," I say.

"Yes! A really good one!"

We receive no direct contact from Lilly after the new security system is installed, and in April of the following year, I become a father when my first son, Robert is born. To celebrate the occasion, my parents fly in from their retirement home in Florida, and Astrid's family comes in from Puerto Rico. My sister, Mary, who is a religious missionary in Brazil, arranges to return to the States so she can perform the christening, and my older brother, Richard, who usually never leaves New York City, drives up in his vintage Cadillac to celebrate the occasion. Many of our friends from the city, my colleagues from the Medical College and the VA, and Astrid's associates from the NLRB in Hartford as well as several of our neighbors also attend. It's a big event.

With the champagne pouring and the party in full swing, I notice a noise that sounds like one of the stereo's speakers is buzzing. Annoyed, I set out to find the defective speaker, but even after switching off all of the sound faders, I notice that the noise hasn't gone away. Instead, it's just become more pronounced. Taking a moment to glance around the room, I realize that the sound isn't coming from inside the house.

Rushing to the front window in panic, I see a little red car with Lilly in the driver's seat. I immediately find Astrid, who is enjoying a conversation with one of her NLRB buddies, pull her aside, and whisper, "She's here."

"Who's here?" she asks, confused.

"Lilly!" I whisper.

"Lilly?" she repeats, confused.

Then it hits her. *Lilly*.

Her expression darkens.

"Where is she?"

"Out in front in her car, and she has been on her horn for a while."

Astrid marches toward the window and pulls the curtain back. The horn is still blaring.

"Go out and get her to stop that noise. I've had enough! I'm calling the police!"

With Astrid on the phone with 911, I confront Lilly. She continues pressing on the horn until I'm standing beside the driver's side window. Seeing me, she takes her hand off the horn and rolls the window down.

"Lilly, you have to leave," I order.

She stares at me and doesn't respond. Looking at her closely, I see that her pupils are dilated with a maniacal intensity that I've only witnessed with patients who are in the throes of a psychosis[10] or using drugs. I also notice that her hair and clothes are disheveled. It appears that she may have been living out of her car for quite some time.

Lilly's eyes turn to Astrid who's outside onto the front steps with the phone in her hand speaking with the 911 operator.

"That bitch!" she utters in an unearthly voice before pressing down on the car horn again.

Worrying that Lilly might further lose control and possibly get out of her car and try to hurt Astrid, I step closer to her car door.

"Lilly, stop! You are causing a disturbance, and we have called the police."

Her eyes turn wild. She looks at me, then at Astrid, and begins screaming incoherently. Still pressing on the horn, she peels out of the driveway like a NASCAR driver. At first, it appears that Lilly's trying to flee the police, but instead of going down the street, she makes a sharp right turn into our driveway and runs straight into the back of my brother's

---

10. Psychosis is a mental state in which a person's thought, emotions and behavior are so impaired by delusions, hallucinations, or agitation that they have lost contact with external reality.

Coupe de Ville, which has a large chrome rear bumper. The resulting impact causes little damage to his Cadillac, but it crumples her car's front hood.

Shifting into reverse, she backs out of the driveway onto our cul-de-sac and roars down the street, the end of which is now blocked by a West Hartford police car with flashing lights. Fortunately, Lilly stops and doesn't crash into the police cruiser. She is immediately arrested and placed in the back of the police car.

Instead of feeling relief, I feel like a failure. *You were her therapist. You failed spectacularly with her; you need to make sure she's alright.*

I walk down the street toward the police and speak with the officers.

"Officers thank you for responding so quickly. I am a psychologist with the VA, and she is one of my patients. She is having a psychiatric emergency and needs to be taken to the VA emergency room. If you will take her there, I will call ahead and arrange for her to be admitted," I say, flashing them my ID.

The two police officers are reluctant to follow my instructions, but the older one returns to the police car and looks at Lilly who is now slumped over in the back seat. After a moment, he turns to me, giving a sympathetic smile and nods.

I return to the house relieved and ready to explain to Astrid that the police are taking Lilly to the hospital. She agrees that it's in Lilly's best interest to get the help that she needs, but I can tell by her body language that she's angry that the situation has gotten this far.

"Just as long as she isn't out there walking around and doesn't come back here!" She warns, before returning to the guests who thankfully are oblivious to the drama that has just transpired. The only exception being my brother who, after we examine his car for damage and find it doesn't have a scratch, says, "And that's why I drive a Cadillac!"

With Astrid happily tending to the guests again, I step out of the room and call the ER at the VA. The night shift nurse picks up the phone but doesn't know me personally. When I identify myself as a psychiatric consultant who works closely on crisis admissions with Dr. Dominick, she becomes cooperative. I briefly explain the details of what occurred and give her my clinical observation of Lilly's condition.

"I believe that she is having a psychotic break and will need to be admitted for observation. I will confer with Dr. Dominick first thing in the morning."

The nurse asks a few more questions and eventually agrees to take care of Lilly's admission when the police arrive.

The situation is far from ideal, but at least I can enjoy the rest of the evening with Astrid and our guests.

~

Psychiatric Shelter
New Britain, Connecticut, 1984

My plan is to meet with both Dr. Daniels and Dr. Dominick to discuss Lilly when they arrive at the VA, but first I have to attend an administrative meeting at the community mental health agency for my side job directing their psychiatric shelter. The agency is housed in an old three-story Victorian mansion, and both my office and the shelter are located on the third floor. Arriving early to prepare, I glance out of the office window at the building's driveway three stories below, and my heart immediately begins to pound in my chest. Lilly's little– and now damaged–red car is sitting there idling.

My mind explodes in confusion. *How can this be? How can she be here? She should be in the hospital. Something is very wrong!*

Leaping down the three flights of stairs, I burst out of the building's side door. Lilly, still looking as disheveled and ragged as she did the night before, is sitting in the driver's seat with the window down.

Bewildered, I ask, "Lilly, what are you doing here?"

With the same wild, maniacal look in her eyes, which are now reddened from lack of sleep, she shouts, "You know why! We are supposed to be together, and that bitch is trying to stop us, so I am going to kill her!"

Kill her…

A nauseating feeling arises within me.

Oh my god! This isn't over. She's going to hurt Astrid.

Instinctively, I reach for the door handle of the car to drag her out and stop her, but before I can, she puts her car in reverse, spins its wheels on the gravel driveway, and turns up the street toward the freeway entrance.

My body is filled with fear as I force myself to run up the three flights of stairs to call Astrid, who is home with our son on maternity leave. Gasping for air, I utter the most outlandish thing I have ever had to say to her in our 50-year relationship.

"Honey, Lilly is not in the hospital. I don't know what happened, but she was just here, and now she's gone! She says she is coming to kill you. I'm calling the police and am on my way."

"Let her try! I've had enough of this woman!" she replies in full mama bear mode.

Frantically hanging up the phone, I call the West Hartford Police Department and then drive home well over the speed limit scanning my surroundings for signs of Lilly. Any woman with dark hair. Any red car. Any erratic behavior. *Somehow, someway, I have to stop her.*

When I pull into my driveway, I look for signs of disturbance or the damaged red car, but, to my relief, everything appears normal. Astrid greets me at the door holding Robert in her arms.

"She hasn't been here, and she'd better not show up! What happened? I thought you were having her hospitalized."

Giving them both a hug, I reply, "I don't know what happened. She just showed up at the shelter. There has clearly been some kind of screw up. I'm going to call Dr. Daniels and find out."

However, before I am able to make the call, the police arrive. After explaining to them what transpired over the past 24 hours, they agree to leave a patrol car in front of our house and issue an all-points bulletin[11] for Lilly.

I call Dr. Daniels after the police leave, and I can hear him becoming upset.

"Let me call Dr. Dominick and find out what the hell happened! I will call you as soon as I know anything. Stay safe!" he shouts.

An hour later Dr. Daniels calls me back clearly still very frustrated.

"Bob, there was a major screw up. According to Dr. Dominick, who is also pissed, the nurse you talked with went off shift before Lilly and the West Hartford police arrived and did not give the information you gave her to the new ER charge nurse at the change of shift meeting. When Lilly arrived at the ER, she apparently presented as calm and lucid and, since they had no other history on her, after a brief evaluation, they

---

11. An *all-points bulletin* is a general notice broadcast to alert law-enforcement officers over a wide area that someone (such as a suspect) or something (such as a vehicle) is being actively sought in connection with a crime.

released her with instructions to check in with the outpatient clinic in the morning."

Great, Lilly is roaming the streets free to do anything she pleases.

The police stay until late evening, but when Lilly doesn't appear, they leave, telling me that they will increase their patrols on our street for the next few weeks.

Astrid and I spend an uneasy but thankfully uneventful evening together.

After a few days without any unusual activity, the tension between us starts to pass. That is, until the phone rings. Astrid and I both look at each other as I pick up the receiver.

"Hello?"

"Bob, it's Dr. Daniels."

Oh, thank heavens! It's not Lilly.

"I was just contacted by a social worker from Connecticut Valley State Hospital. Apparently, the state police picked up Lilly on the interstate after she left you due to her erratic driving, and after assessing her mental state, they brought her to the hospital to have her committed."

Glancing at Astrid, I cover the phone and whisper, "It's Dr. Daniels. Lilly is in the state hospital." We both smile at the news.

"The social worker from the state hospital wanted to transfer her to us here at the VA. I declined, telling them that I felt she was too hot for us to handle, especially after what she put you and your wife through," Dr. Daniels adds sardonically.

Any beliefs that I had about being able to help Lilly have long dissipated, and I don't give Dr. Daniels any resistance.

～

It takes some time for my emotions to settle. I feel guilty over what I've put Astrid through. She has every right to be angry with me for how I've mishandled the situation, but I'm grateful that, in time, she decides to forgive me. There's a renewed sense of understanding on my part, though, that my profession carries certain risks and that I am responsible for recognizing and managing them.

I also continue to struggle with how naïve I was about Lilly's condition. She was clearly suffering from episodes of depression, which is what I focused on in her treatment, but the significance of her unstable and emotionally exaggerated behaviors, I completely missed.

While many of Lilly's symptoms are consistent with borderline personality disorder (BPD), this label does not meet the criteria for an accurate and complete diagnosis. At its core, this disorder involves an intense fear of abandonment and the tendency to overreact to interpersonal loss—both real and perceived. This disease can also distort the patient's thinking as well as their emotional and behavioral reactions. Delusional thinking, however, is not a primary symptom of the disorder. It was Lilly's delusional[12] belief about the nature of our relationship that drove her violation of the fourth wall.

The specific type of delusion that's more consistent with Lilly's symptoms is a disorder known as Erotomania or "delusional love" (a condition that was first defined in France in the late 19th century by the psychiatrist Gaëtan de Clérambault). It is also known as Clérambault's Syndrome—a subtype of delu-

---

12. Delusions are fixed (persistent), false beliefs regarding the self or other persons or objects outside the self that conflict with reality and are maintained despite indisputable evidence to the contrary.

sion disorders in the most recent edition of American Psychiatric Association's diagnostic manual[13].

Erotomania is characterized by an individual's fixation on another person as their lover, romantic partner, or the object of their sexual desire despite the absence of evidence of a romantic relationship. The object of this infatuation is typically unaware of the situation and the person's emotional attachment to them, causing the patient to become obsessed, even aggressive, in their attempts to communicate with them. This disorder can also coexist with other disorders, like depression, making it more difficult to diagnose.

With this disorder, however, there are never any hallucinations. This is why Lilly was able to present herself as lucid at the hospital.

~

New Berlin, Connecticut, 1985

While Lilly never threatened us again, I did run into her a year later. I had taken a second part-time job directing a psychosocial rehabilitation program[14] for recently discharged patients in a neighboring town, and the position involved supervising the staff involved in prevocational work training, educational, and social support services. It was also my role to screen clients for the program.

---

13. American Psychiatric Association. *Diagnostic and Statistical Manual of Mental Disorders* (5th ed.; DSM-5); pg. 90-93.

14. A psychosocial rehabilitation program focuses on helping individuals with mental illness regain and improve essential social and vocational skills to enhance their quality of life and functioning within the community. This approach can help individuals return to work or school and achieve greater independence.

One day, the program secretary buzzed me to announce that there was a new female client in the waiting room. Looking down at the one-page admission form, which was mostly empty except for the patient's name, sex, age, date of birth, and marital status, I noted that the person was divorced and had been discharged from the state hospital. Thinking I would acquire more information during the interview, I headed to the waiting room to meet the patient.

Sitting in a chair near the door was a casually dressed and neatly groomed woman with dark hair reading a magazine. As I approached her, she looked up and we made eye contact. My mouth suddenly went dry with the taste of fear as I recognized that, while she didn't look as crazed and disheveled as when I last saw her, it was definitely Lilly. The reason I didn't recognize her name on the intake form was because she had divorced her husband, Charles, and was using her maiden name. Her middle name Lilly, short for Lilith, was also not on the form.

Shocked, I didn't know whether to admit her or send her packing. Thankfully, Lilly answered all of those questions for me. Once she recognized me, she stood up, dropped the magazine, screamed, and ran out of the building.

After that, I never saw her again, and, to my great relief, she never attempted to contact me or Astrid.

Surviving this ordeal with Astrid strengthened the bonds of our relationship. While we rarely talk about Lilly now, when she does come up in conversation, I'm always struck by the differences in our emotional recollection of the events. I remember feeling a sense of helplessness and fear as the true nature of Lilly's psychological disturbance revealed itself, but Astrid's memories are quite different.

"At the time, I don't recall ever being scared of that woman. Angry, yes, but scared, no," she recalled. "For me, she was a problem to be dealt with. She threatened our family, and I never had any doubt about my ability to protect our family. I knew that for you it was more complicated because you were her doctor, but for me it was simple. No one threatens my family! When I think about her now, though, I feel sorry for her. She was clearly suffering."

The situation was indeed more complicated for me. I was Lilly's psychotherapist and had a duty to act in her best interest. Even though, as Dr. Daniels observed in supervision, her actions prevented me from executing my role, I still felt guilty for years over how my lack of awareness contributed to this situation.

This was, however, an important, if not humbling and cautionary, learning experience for me about the complex and powerful dynamics of the psychotherapeutic relationship between patient and doctor—one that made me painfully aware of the traumatic consequences of any violation of the fourth wall of the treatment office. These consequences still linger with me to this day so much so that when I see a small red car with some body damage, my heart rate increases slightly and the hair on the back of my neck stands up.

Questions for Consideration

1. If you were in the author's situation, how would you pick up on the signs that he missed? What do you believe he did wrong in this situation?
2. What do you think triggered Lilly's romantic feelings, causing her to develop an unhealthy

attachment to her therapist? Do you believe that she lacked a father figure or something else?

3. How did the author cope with this emotional trauma? How would you cope if you were in a similar situation that impacted not just you but your family?

4. In the modern day, stalking can take on many forms such as cyberstalking. How would you handle stalking now versus how the author handled it then?

5. If you were the spouse in this situation, how do you think you would have handled or communicated your feelings?

6. How could the author have avoided the mistake that occurred with the night shift nurse? What could have been done differently then and now?

7. Why did Dr. Daniels have to intervene? Why couldn't the author see that there were significant challenges with Lilly and that he couldn't treat her?

8. Would medication in this circumstance be helpful in treating an unhealthy attraction to a therapist?

9. Do you think that therapists and academics are particularly vulnerable to erotomania? Why?

THE FORGETFUL BAGMAN

VA Medical Center
Newington, Connecticut, 1985

"Bob, I would like you to treat a patient whom I think you'll find interesting. He's suffering from some kind of panic disorder but is also apparently having some memory issues. It should only require a brief course of treatment, and I think you can wrap it up before you leave."

Still in the throes of winter this bitterly cold February morning, I sit in Dr. Daniels' office still celebrating the defense of my dissertation and completion of my PhD program. I've just been offered a postdoctoral residency in neuropsychology and trauma that will begin in July at a community mental health center in southern Massachusetts. Focused on wrapping up my clinical work, completing treatment with patients, and transferring the remaining ones to other clinicians, I know that taking on a new case will be difficult, but Dr. Daniels has been a great mentor and friend, so I agree to do it.

When I meet, Tony[1], a short, heavyset man in his late fifties for our first session, I start the conversation with a basic question.

"What brings you here, Tony? I understand you've been in the ER a couple of times recently."

Staring at his hands, he flexes his fingers nervously.

"Yeah, it's been weekly as of late. I don't understand what's happening to me. I keep having these episodes where my heart suddenly starts racing. Then I can't breathe, my vision gets all blurry, and I feel like I am going to pass out."

"How long has this been happening to you?" I ask.

"It started this last year, a few months after I had the operation on this bum ticker[2]," he says, pointing to his chest. "The heart doctor says that when I have these episodes, it could be another heart attack and that I should go to the ER and be evaluated. However, every time I go, they do a workup and tell me it's not my heart. They say it's stress and that I'm having panic attacks. The last time I was in the ER, they gave me some pills—Xanax, I think—and made an appointment for me to come here."

Looking embarrassed, Tony adds, "I've never had anything like this happen before. Not even during the war and that was

---

1. Name has been changed
2. Bum ticker: a bad heart

pretty stressful. Sometimes when this happens, I feel like I'm going crazy and losing control."

"Sounds like the episodes are pretty scary. Does anything specific trigger them?" I ask.

Tony slumps over in the chair, takes a deep breath, and swallows hard. I can see that he is trying to choke back an intense emotion.

"Well, I can tell you it ain't no picnic. And it's getting in the way of things," he replies, gritting his teeth before slipping into silence.

I'm immediately struck by a feeling of guardedness. While he doesn't present as hostile or defensive about the nature of his panic attacks, he's unusually vague about the circumstances that trigger them and other aspects of his personal history. His sarcastic tone isn't helping either, but I know that he isn't referring to me or the therapeutic process. He's clearly terrified and helpless about something else altogether, and his panic attacks are getting in the way of it. *But what?*

As we sit in silence for close to an hour, Tony has completely withdrawn into himself and looks emotionally exhausted. Recognizing that nothing else will be accomplished today, I make the executive decision to end the session.

"I can see that this has been very difficult for you. I would like to continue exploring this during our next session, and I believe that if we work together, you can get control of what's happening to you."

"You really think so, Doc?" he asks bewildered at the suggestion.

"Yes, Tony, I definitely do," I reply, masking my concern with confidence.

～

When a patient is guarded in psychotherapy, the underlying issue is trust. Even though the patient knows that they're in a medical setting, the psychotherapist is still just a stranger to them. One of my colleagues once observed that in medical settings, physicians and nurses have an advantage over psychologists because they wear white coats with stethoscopes draped around their neck, which gives them an air of authority and identifies their role, while psychologists wear civilian clothes, which can make their function appear more ambiguous[3]. Standing out in a clearly defined role is the exact opposite of what I learned as an investigator on the streets of New York City. Blending in was an essential part of not just the job but survival itself. Interestingly, Tony's tracksuit was the outfit of choice of some of the people I investigated as a fed.

Since building trust is the first step in establishing a stable therapeutic alliance [4], it's important to make Tony feel comfortable. I start by slowly introducing and familiarizing him to the psychotherapeutic process so that it's less intimidating for him. One key strategy is to make each session feel conversational rather than interrogational.

During our next session, Tony appears more relaxed as he settles into the leather chair in my office. He's almost a bit chatty.

"How are things going, Tony?"

"Okay, Doc. I haven't had any panic attacks since our last session."

---

3. In the mid 1980s, most psychologist at Newington, including me, wore sports jackets and ties when treating patients.

4. The therapeutic alliance refers to the collaborative relationship between a client and therapist, which plays a central role in effective psychotherapy.

"That's great!"

Given his guardedness and my concern about the fragile nature of our treatment alliance, I decide not to immediately probe into the circumstances surrounding his panic attacks. Instead, I begin by asking some general background questions about his family, upbringing, education, relationship status, and military career. Since he has already provided some of this information on the intake forms, I feel he will be comfortable sharing it.

"So, Tony, tell me a bit about yourself. Are you from around here?" I ask casually.

"My family has been in this part of Connecticut for a while. They came up here from Bridgeport in the late 30s. When I was a kid growing up here in the 40s during World War II, my parents and everybody else I knew worked in the factories around here."

"What was it like growing up here?"

"You might say I grew up in the rough part of town. All us kids in the neighborhood were in gangs. It was a matter of survival. There were lots of fights, so, you had to be in one if you didn't want to get beat up all the time. Anyway, when I got out of high school, it was in the early 1950s. I was 18 and immediately got drafted into the Army and sent to Korea."

"What was it like being in the Army in Korea?"

He pauses for a moment and rubs his eyes.

"I was a grunt[5]. Ended up on the front lines, so I saw a lot of action. Those human wave assaults were pretty crazy. A bunch of guys screaming and running at you. Sometimes without any bullets, just rifles with bayonets."

Thinking that maybe post-traumatic stress from the war

---

5. Grunt: a low-ranking or unskilled soldier

could be playing a role in his panic episodes, I decide to probe this a bit more.

"Do you think about being in the war much?"

"Nah. To be honest, it wasn't much worse than some of the fights and shootings I'd seen in the streets here growing up—just more of it. No, I don't think about that war much at all."

Strike one, but I do notice a brightness on his face.

"Actually, Doc, I liked being in the Army. It was predictable, and if you followed the rules, no one messed with you. Also, you got fed regularly, which wasn't always true at home when I was a kid. Stayed in for two more tours after coming back from Korea."

He seems willing to talk about his military experience, so I continue to explore this further.

"Why did you leave?" I ask.

"I started to miss my family and my old friends back in the neighborhood, so I didn't re-up after my second tour and came back home. Got married to my old girlfriend, Anita, and hooked back up with my old gang. Picked up doin' what I'd been doin' with them before I got drafted. It was like I'd never left."

Tony's chatty demeanor suddenly changes. He sits back in his chair and looks out the window. Recalling that he listed "messenger" as his job on his intake form, I have a hunch that his gang-related activities may be related to his panic attacks, but he's not ready to talk yet, so I let silence do the work.

A month into his treatment, Tony's cagey demeanor about his job starts to crack. His panic attacks have started to increase again, and under their looming pressure, he decides to open up, but he wants a few assurances first.

"Doc, all this stuff we talk about in here, it's confidential, right? Like, you can't tell nobody, right? You know like when you tell a lawyer something you did?" he says while his knees bounce up and down.

Of course, I had explained the nature of our confidentiality agreement at the beginning of his treatment, as I routinely do with all my patients, but there is an uncertainty in his question that feels familiar. Suddenly, I remember what my boss Charlie Annibale told me about dealing with informants. *Bob, whatever their motivation, informants are taking a big risk in talking with you. So, you have to constantly reassure them that no one is going to find out about it. It's the key to getting information from them.*

Thinking about his advice, I try to reassure Tony.

"Tony, for therapy to work you have to feel comfortable telling me everything about your condition and situation, and, to do that, you have to be able to trust that I'm not going to tell anyone else what you say. Because of this, I am ethically and legally bound not to reveal anything that you tell me. There are some very limited exceptions for safety, like if you tell me that you are going to harm yourself or someone else, but, even then, I can only divulge what's necessary to protect you and others."

"Well, this ain't about that kind of stuff. I ain't about to harm anybody. I don't do the rough stuff no more," he adds cryptically. "But I'm worried about me getting done by somebody else. So, you can't talk, right?"

"That's right, Tony. I can't talk."

Tony clasps his hands together and exhales.

"Like I said, Doc, when I got back home, I just sort of picked up with the guys where I left off before I went into the Army. Only now, they were more organized about it, and there was also a lot more money involved, which was where my having been a soldier in the war came in useful."

As my investigative background fills in the blanks, it

becomes clear that his childhood friends—the guys—are the local mob and that "picking up where he'd left off" involves a range of illegal activities including gambling, bookmaking, and loan sharking. The usefulness of his war experience makes him a street-level enforcer.

"My crew had the gambling business—booking bets on the ponies and sports, especially football, and loaning money out to local guys who couldn't deal with the banks. We didn't deal with drugs or the girls. Other crews had that business."

He pauses, rubbing his palms against his legs.

"Didn't like doin' the rough stuff. I avoided it when I could, but sometimes if somebody wasn't paying up, it was necessary. Didn't do nothin' serious, though. Nothin' like whacking somebody or anything like that. Other guys did that stuff. After a while, I was mostly a bagman[6]. You know, collecting the money from the bookies and payments on the loans, passing it on to the bosses, and delivering payoffs to other people. You'd be surprised who was on the take."

He adds that he had been arrested a few times but was never convicted of anything or went to jail for any of his "activities."

"Evidence would disappear and witnesses didn't show up to testify," he explains. "Hell, sometimes the cops didn't even show up at the hearings."

Listening to Tony's description of his world reminds me of a few individuals in the mob that I investigated working for Charlie and the agency in New York. Some were pure psychopaths—dangerous, with no empathy and prone to violence—but others, like Tony, were guys who had grown up in a world where the rules weren't so black and white. These

---

6. Bagman: someone who collects or delivers illegal payments or illegally earned money for someone else.

individuals were neither dangerous nor particularly violent, and I often found them quite charming and unassuming.

"Things were okay until my ticker started going bad," he continues. "I was in my early fifties. Kept getting these chest pains when I'd get physical with someone. After a while, it was clear that I wasn't going to be able to do the rough stuff anymore. So, the bosses just had me doin' the collections. I became a bagman full time. Spent my days driving around picking up and dropping off money at different locations. Kind of liked the job. It was low stress, but one thing you needed to do was to keep the details about the money in order. You had to remember who got what and how much. That was very important 'cause if you messed up the money, there'd be serious consequences, and that's where my problems really began, Doc."

While his cardiologist initially managed his condition with medications, Tony suffered multiple heart attacks due to several blocked arteries and weakened heart valves and had to have open heart surgery.

"After the surgery, I kept getting things all mixed up. I couldn't remember the amounts accurately or who gave me what or when or where. I started making mistakes."

I nod, understanding the severity of his situation.

"And in my world, if you make mistakes with the money, the bosses get unhappy, and when the bosses get unhappy, bad things happen to you."

Tony's comment triggers a memory of one of Charlie Annibale's lessons to me about the mob after the attempted hit: *They're dangerous especially when money is involved, and we messed with their money. And you don't mess with their money. Violence to them is just another tool, and they use it with about as much feeling.*

Images of my car sliding off the New Jersey turnpike flash

through my mind, and a shiver runs down my spine. I've struggled for years with the idea that someone purposely tried to kill me and the fear that they might try again. As these emotions flood my consciousness, I understand—no, actually feel—the terror that Tony is experiencing.

Tony's complaints of memory loss remind me of the late 1970s and the early 1980s when, depending on where a patient's cardiac operation was performed, they were at risk for brain damage post-surgery. This was because the cardiopulmonary (heart/lung) bypass pumps of the time were inefficient. Open-heart patients sometimes suffered a temporary loss of oxygen to the brain, referred to as anoxia, during the procedure. This caused neurons[7] in the brain to die resulting in a loss of brain function. It was not uncommon during this time for patients to complain of short-term memory, attention, and concentration problems.

Suspicious that this might be what happened to Tony given the timing of his heart operation, I decide to consult Dr. Daniels about his condition. He agrees that Tony's cognitive symptoms seem consistent with the presence of anoxic brain damage.

"Dan, I think the best way to fully assess this problem

---

7. Neurons are the primary cells in the nervous system responsible for relaying information, coordinating bodily functions, and enabling cognitive processes.

would be to do a full neuropsychological evaluation[8] and for him to have a CAT scan[9]."

"I agree, Bob. A neuropsychological evaluation is the way to go here. I will see about getting him a CAT scan at the Medical College. What about his panic symptoms?"

"I want to hold off on any medications until after the neuropsychological evaluation, but I will begin teaching him breathing and relaxation techniques that should help in the meantime. If I am right about the test results, I have an idea that might eliminate his symptoms without needing to use medication."

Excited about the idea, I head to my office and wait for Tony. After he settles in, I make my proposal.

"Tony, based on everything you've told me, I'd like to do some testing to find out how severe your problems with memory and attention really are. I'd also like you to have a brain scan at the medical college."

"Doc, if you think that's what I need to do, I'm okay with it," he says without any resistance.

I schedule his neuropsychological evaluation with me, and

---

8. A neuropsychological evaluation is an extensive battery of tests designed to compare a patient's current cognitive functioning with their estimated prior level of functioning and that of others their age. These tests are cognitive experiments that measure among other things memory, attention, concentration, judgment, and problem solving. Once the data on the various cognitive functions is collected, statistical analysis is then used to measure variations in performance from the expected norms. If the patient's performance is significantly below what would be statistically expected, it suggests the presence of a cognitive deficit. However, while these tests can indicate the presence of a deficit, the actual cause of the deficit can only be determined from the patient's clinical history and information on their neuroanatomy (i.e., data that can be obtained from an X-ray, MRI or CAT scan.

9. MRIs, which I would recommend today, were not readily available at the time.

Dr. Daniels pulls in a favor and prepares his CAT scan at the Medical College for the following week.

The results are what I expected. The neuropsychological testing indicates that while he is still of average global intelligence, he's exhibiting specific neurocognitive deficits[10] that are interfering with his functioning. Most notably, in relation to others his age, his brain's capacity to focus on and retain new information, especially numerical information is impaired.

This data is consistent with the findings from his CAT scan, which reveal the presence of mild but widespread atrophy across his neocortex[11]. Unlike a stroke or a concussion, which causes damage to a specific area of the brain, the negative effects of oxygen deprivation are much broader and affect most of the brain's neurons. Taken together, this pattern is consistent with the cerebral anoxia associated with the faulty heart/lung bypass pumps used in his cardiac surgery.

With the evaluation and CAT data in hand, I focus on getting Tony to understand the connection between his panic attacks, as they are the result of his growing fear of his bosses and what they might do to him if he continues messing up cash drops, and the cognitive symptoms that are a side effect of his cardiac surgery. However, I have to translate complex neuropsychological and medical information into a language he can understand and use.

---

10. Neurocognitive deficits refer to impairments in the brain's cognitive functions such as memory, attention, problem-solving, and perception due to a medical disease other than a psychiatric illness.

11. Neocortex atrophy refers to the loss of neurons and the reduction in size of the neocortex, which is the outermost layer of the cerebral cortex responsible for higher cognitive functions.

The results of a neuropsychological evaluation usually have two audiences: one is a professional audience made up of neuropsychologists, neurologists, psychiatrists, physicians, and nurses, and the second is the patient and their family. The first group requires a significant amount of technical detail and analysis for the information to be useful to them. For the second group, however, such technical information is not always necessary or beneficial.

For this latter group, part of the job involves being able to translate clinical data into everyday language. This is why I use a 3-D plastic model of the brain to teach my patients. It turns abstract concepts into concrete reality.

It's important to note, however, that sharing this information with the patient can cause emotional distress. This is especially true in Tony's case given the terror that's driving his panic attacks. Once I'm satisfied that he understands my explanation of the findings, we then explore how best to approach the situation with his mob bosses.

"Sometimes, the bosses, they just don't want to listen, and then bad things happen," he admits.

My concern for Tony's well-being increases. It's not enough for him to understand his cognitive deficits. We're going to have to orchestrate a plan that he can execute outside the safety of my office so that 'bad things' won't happen to him.

"You know, Doc, I've been thinking about how to present all this to my bosses," he says during our next treatment session. "If you write a short summary on official VA letterhead with a government seal explaining that my heart surgery is causing me to have trouble remembering things, they just might understand."

"That's a great idea, Tony. Let's work on it together," I say, feeling a sense of relief.

After I draft a preliminary letter, we use our next few sessions to edit and simplify it. Interestingly, while we remove most of the technical medical terms from the letter, Tony insists that we keep some in because he feels it makes the letter sound more official.

Once Tony is satisfied, we role play how he's going to explain this information to his bosses. This is because the world in which Tony operates is so clandestine that it has its own street parlance made up of deliberately vague terms like "That thing I do on Tuesdays with that guy." In some cases, the meaning of the slang he's using is totally obscure to me, but I have to trust the process. After a few practice rounds, he seems satisfied with his presentation and feels ready to approach his bosses.

~

I sit in my office tapping my feet as I anxiously wait for Tony to come through my office door for our next therapy session. Knowing from experience how the bosses in his world operate, I find myself thinking, *What if his bosses don't believe him—or worse—don't care enough to listen?* I am concerned that there's a good possibility that he won't walk through that door ever again, the implications of which I can't bear to imagine.

Trying to allay my anxiety, I busy myself with paperwork when suddenly I hear a knock at the door. Tony enters my office looking relieved and reassured. Gone is the terrified man that came into my office suffering from chronic panic attacks. He's happy, talkative, and jovial!

"Well, how did it go?" I blurt out unable to contain my excitement.

"Surprisingly well, Doc," he says, smiling. "They actually seemed very interested in the medical stuff. Who would've thought? Anyway, they said they had noticed I was having trouble with the money and now that they knew what the problem was, I don' have to pick the money up anymore. I just drive somebody else, and he gets the money."

A simple yet elegant solution.

I continued to work with Tony for several more treatment sessions but after he presented the letter to his bosses, his panic attacks ceased almost immediately. However, he liked the breathing and relaxation techniques he'd been practicing and wanted to learn more.

During our last session, Tony presented me with a hand-crocheted bookmark with the word *Doc* embroidered in red.

"I had my wife do it for me, Doc. She likes doing this kind of thing and says it relaxes her. You saved my neck, Doc, and I wanted to give you something to remember me by. I know you can't accept expensive gifts, so I hope this is okay."

"It's perfect, Tony," I say, moved by his sweet gesture.

Over the course of my career, I've had numerous opportunities to treat patients who were known for being the dangerous "tough guys." But interestingly, these individuals almost always had a softer side.

"Oh, and Doc, I'm getting out of the business here. Sort of retiring. You know my health and all. I know some guys in Vegas. They tell me the climate there will be much better for my health than the climate here. So, me and the wife are moving there. Kind of a new beginning."

Given the unusual double speak of Tony's street language, I'm not quite sure whether "climate" refers to the weather or something more unsettling concerning his career path.

"Sounds like a good plan, Tony. However, with your heart and everything, you might need more care. I'll ask the clinic secretary to get you information on the VA medical center there, and we can make referrals if you want. Good luck with the move."

"You too, Doc," he says, shaking my hand before leaving my office for the last time.

Tony was the last patient that Dr. Daniels referred to me while I was in training under him. Although he couched it as me doing a favor for him, I believe that he knew that Tony would teach me something I needed to know as a psychotherapist. He was right.

What I learned early on in my career is that one cannot simply be a psychotherapist by reading books. It's a lived, intimate, and interpersonal experience—one that touches every part of the human soul, including personal beliefs, life experiences, and even prejudices. These emotional reactions on part of the psychotherapist, known as countertransference[12], must be recognized early on and controlled if a patient is to receive effective treatment.

In working through these emotions with Dr. Daniels over the past four years, we discussed many aspects of my life and relationships including the trauma of the accident on the New Jersey Turnpike that led to my decision to change my career. Just as he felt that I had needed to work through my feelings

---

12. Countertransference refers to the therapist's conscious or unconscious reactions to a patient. These reactions may include thoughts and feelings and are shaped by the therapist's own psychological needs and conflicts that are activated in the therapeutic relationship. The complementary concept, transference, originally coined in psychoanalysis, describes the patient's unconscious redirection of feelings and wishes—originally directed toward significant figures such as parents in childhood—onto the therapist. Today, the term is used more broadly to refer to a patient's emotional responses, positive or negative, toward the therapist.

around the Vietnam War to effectively treat Billy, I believe that he referred Tony to me because he knew that I needed to process an entirely different set of emotions.

Working with Tony brought back memories, not just of the accident, but of other dealings I had as a government investigator. While these experiences gave me insight about Tony that was useful in his treatment, some of the emotions that were stirred up in me, especially the ones connected to violence, were very disturbing. However, the success of Tony's treatment was in seeing him not as a low-level gangster but as a fellow human being who was frightened and suffering. That allowed me to ultimately overcome my own thoughts and feelings by returning to the dark world I thought I'd left years before.

Tony was also the first person that I treated after receiving my doctorate. While I was still in training during my residency, I was now referred to by patients and colleagues as *Dr.* Gillespie. The title came with a new set of expectations and responsibilities, but I felt an increased sense of freedom in my treatment approach that allowed me to be more experimental, especially with my knowledge as an investigator.

In the world of practicing neuropsychologists, there are two groups of clinicians. By far the largest group are those solely focused on the assessment process. They spend many hours with patients learning their history and sometimes meet with the patient's significant others to collect additional information, but they don't actually treat the patient. Their involvement ends with giving the patient feedback on the test results and writing a report that goes to a physician or other clinician. In this regard, they are more like radiologists who look at the scan and interpret it but don't actually treat the patient's condition.

The second group do what I call *applied* neuropsychology.

They conduct the same evaluations but then take the information and integrate it with other clinical and neuroscientific data. This is done to treat the patient and improve their functioning rather than simply assign them a diagnostic label. Taking dry medical data and crafting it into an action plan for Tony to use outside the safety of my office placed me squarely in the applied neuropsychology camp.

Questions for Consideration

1. In this circumstance, how would you have gauged Tony's well-being, considering he was reserved and guarded at the onset?
2. What were identifiable traits (i.e., characteristics and behaviors) that revealed that Tony's well-being had been compromised?
3. What did the author do well to gain this patient's trust? Would you have done the same? Is there anything you would have done differently?
4. Is it possible that if the author had continued the first session without ending it, it would have compromised the therapeutic alliance?
5. Do you think it would have been beneficial to be heavier handed with Tony, especially since the author was leaving the organization and his time was limited? Do you think Tony would have had the same experience if he had been transferred to another doctor?
6. Give defined examples that the therapist used to gain Tony's trust that ultimately allowed him to open up. How did the author exceed expectations?

7. How did the author's training at the agency help him in this situation?

8. Do you believe Dr. Daniels acted as an assessment psychologist by assigning the author this patient? Do you think that Dr. Daniels treated the author so that the author could treat the patient?

THE ANGUISHED SNIPER

— IRVIN D. YALOM, 1995

VA Medical Center
Newington, Connecticut, 1985

As I sit at my desk processing admissions forms, my colleague and friend, Dr. Larry Baker, wanders into my office and plunks himself down in a vacant chair. He glances at the piles of file boxes, books, and papers in front me while I scribble notes finalizing the last details of my caseloads before leaving Newington for good.

Larry is a fellow psychologist at the clinic. We first met during my internship and have become good friends over the past four years. He was also a member of the research team at the medical college and had been instrumental in our study of relapse rates.

As he lounges in the office chair with one leg drooped over an armrest idly fidgeting with one of my pens, I can tell he is bursting to tell me something.

"Okay, Larry, what is it?" I ask, putting my pen down.

"Dan's retiring! It was just announced at the staff meeting."

"Retiring? When?" I ask, momentarily stunned.

"End of July. That's just after you leave for your residency, isn't it?"

I'm unable to digest that the man who's mentored me for the last four years is retiring.

"Yeah," I say, distractedly before swooping past him toward the hallway and bursting through Dr. Daniels' office without knocking. He's sitting behind his desk reading a journal article.

"You're retiring?" I say, bumfuzzled.

"Yes. It's time. I've been eligible to retire for the past year but wanted to finish some things before I left," he says, looking over his plastic horn-rimmed glasses.

I start to protest, but Dan raises the palm of his hand to stop me.

"Bob, I've been at Newington longer than anybody else besides Helen who, I think, has been here forever. Lately, I've been feeling stagnant, and I am looking to do something new. My wife and I have decided to move to New Mexico. I've gotten licensed there and have found an opportunity to work with the

Indian Health Service. I actually did some work with them as a volunteer during my graduate training at Chapel Hill[1], which was fascinating, and they need mental health services."

Emotionally whiplashed, my thoughts feel paralyzed. Somehow, though, I manage to mumble a proposal for us to go out for dinner so I can give him a proper send-off. Dan and I make plans to meet at the Hartford Hotel, which has one of the better restaurants in town.

The dinner begins awkwardly since we've never socialized outside of a clinical setting, but we eventually discuss his post-retirement plans and my upcoming residency. We also reminisce about our careers over several glasses of pinot noir, the awkwardness fading into nostalgia.

As we speak about the cases we've shared—Billy, Manny, Mike, Tony, and even Lilly—we both feel a sense of profound gratitude for having met each other. Still, a twinge of sadness hangs in the air. The realization that we're parting ways becomes real, and it's clear that our clinical partnership has not only benefited both of us but also created a bond of trust that's just as deep as the unconscious mind.

As I chew my last bite of steak, Dan speaks, causing me to place the white napkin on my plate.

"Bob, I know you're about to start your residency, but I am wondering if you would like to also continue doing the post-traumatic stress group after I retire. I've talked to the Chief of Psychology about it, and he is willing to have you do it if you want to," he says before taking a long sip of wine.

Dan had involved me as a co-therapist in the post-traumatic stress group that he ran on Tuesday nights since I was an intern. Watching him work with the patients was a powerful learning experience for me. It influenced how I practice

---

1. Chapel Hill: The University of North Carolina at Chapel Hill.

psychotherapy in ways that I've still yet to fully comprehend. And now, he's proposing that I become the group's primary therapist—a parting gift that acknowledges my professional growth.

"Dan, it would be a privilege to do it," I say, leaning forward.

As we stand outside the Hartford Hotel, Dan extends his had to say goodbye, and the realization dawns on me that the man who has patiently (and painstakingly) taken a naïve intern and turned him into a psychotherapist is leaving forever. I grasp his hand tightly with both of mine and choke back the tears welling up in my eyes.

"Dan, I really don't know how to thank you for everything you've done for me. Working with you over the past four years has changed me. You have not only shown me what it means to be a psychologist, but, more importantly, you've made me a better therapist. I'm going to miss our conversations."

Dan smiles, looking down at the ground and then at me. True to form, however, he maintains his characteristic reserve and stoicism.

"Bob, it's been a pleasure. Good luck with your residency and the group," he says before walking away into the late spring night.

Six months later, I receive a postcard from New Mexico in which he shares that he's started working part-time with the Indian Health Service and is enjoying it. We exchange Christmas cards for a few years, but as I move around the country, we eventually lose touch.

Three months after I assume the role as the group's primary therapist, my colleague and friend, Dr. Dominick, the head of inpatient psychiatry, contacts me regarding a patient whom he feels could benefit from participating in the group sessions.

The patient, Richard[2], is an ex-marine in his late thirties who's been admitted to the hospital due to a suicide attempt involving drugs and alcohol after he was found by the Hartford police unconscious under a bridge. Dr. Dominick tells me that they know very little about him.

"Bob, we weren't able to get much out of him on the inpatient unit. Wouldn't discuss the suicide attempt or much of anything. From what little we have been able to gather, he has never been in contact with the VA before. He appears to have been homeless for some time, living in a van. The home address on his license is from northern Vermont, and he wouldn't give us any emergency contact information or next of kin. He did say he's been divorced for a long time, and I get the feeling he's been a loner drifting around for a while. He's been quiet and socially withdrawn on the unit but has screaming nightmares almost every night, so he's probably suffering from post-traumatic stress. I've assigned my chief resident to treat him individually, but I think your post-traumatic stress group can also help him."

"Is he still in the hospital? I'd like to meet him," I reply.

"Yes, he's still here. Doesn't seem to have a place to go, so he'll be here for a while until we can work something out for him. I can arrange for you to meet him before your group next week."

As planned, I meet with Richard the following Tuesday evening in an office in the Mental Hygiene Clinic before the start of group. He is a thin and bearded man with a hawkish face dressed in surplus military fatigues. As he enters the

---

2. Name has been changed.

office, I can see his eyes surveying the room looking for a threat.

He then circles the empty chair opposite me before tentatively sitting on its edge. He stares at me so intensely that I start to feel uncomfortable. There's a haunted and feral quality to his expression, as if he's cornered a wild animal and is ready to flee...or pounce.

Overcoming my discomfort, I introduce myself. "Richard, I'm Dr. Gillespie. I'm a psychologist consultant to the VA here at Newington, and Dr. Dominick thinks I might be able to help you."

Since the goal in this meeting is to determine if he's a good fit for the Tuesday night group, given the tension he's exhibiting, I decide not to inquire about his suicide attempt. Instead, I begin with a nonintrusive and innocuous question.

"Tell me a bit about yourself. Where'd you grow up?"

He doesn't respond at first. Instead, he continues sizing me up, looking first at my feet, then slowly moving his gaze up to my knees, stomach, chest, and, finally, my face. Still wary but satisfied that I don't pose a threat, he finally responds in a clipped and flat monotone.

"Little town in Vermont just south of the Canadian border. Not many people. Lived on a farm with my folks. We were poor. Lost the farm when they died."

"Any brothers or sisters?"

"Got an older sister somewhere. She got married and moved away. Haven't heard from her since I enlisted."

"Marines, right?"

His eyes are no longer fixed on me. He's not hunting anymore.

"Yep, joined up in '66. Right out of high school. Going to save the free world from communism. "A few good men" and all that crap. Thought I was gonna be a 30-year man. A lifer, but it didn't work out."

"Vietnam?"

"Yep. That was my war."

"Tough?"

"Yeah," he says before falling silent. I observe as his gaze drifts away from me toward my office window.

In similar situations, I've probed patients with questions like *You seem to be experiencing something. I wonder if you could tell me what you're feeling right now?* But with Richard, my therapeutic instincts tell me that he's psychologically fragile and that any attempt to get him to open up will cause him to shut down or flee.

Also, I've already accomplished the purpose of this interview. Given the way he speaks about his military service combined with his distant stare, and the screaming nightmares Dr. Dominick told me about, he appears to be suffering from post-traumatic stress like the other group members. So, I decide not to inquire further and shift to pitching the idea of group therapy to him.

"Richard, there is a group of Vietnam combat vets that I work with who meet here every Tuesday evening. All of them are struggling with what happened to them over there. They tell me that being with other vets who are going through the same things helps, and I think it might help you, too. I'd like you to consider joining us."

Richard refocuses his attention on me again, but this time his stare is much less feral and more pensive. We sit in silence for another minute as he contemplates the suggestion.

"I don't know, Doc. I'll have to think it over."

~

Since beginning my residency at the community mental health center in southern Massachusetts, I've enjoyed taking the backcountry roads to commute from my home in West Hartford. It provides a 30-minute tranquil drive through beautiful countryside—a transition that is especially helpful on the Tuesday nights since it allows me to mentally prepare to run the group. Tonight, however, as I traverse the tree-lined roads, I'm preoccupied with thoughts of Richard.

Richard has been coming to group for two months since he started psychotherapy, and I can see that he is still struggling. While he seems less apprehensive about being in the group, he hasn't said a word other than when he introduced himself as a marine on the first day. I sense that his prolonged silence is beginning to disturb the other group members. Due to his psychological fragility, I know that I have to tread carefully with him without disrupting the group's ecosystem.

We meet in the same room where the incident between Mike and Dr. M took place, which still carries some traumatic memories for me. The space itself, though, is nondescript with a table and a few chairs used for meetings. Helen, like the angel that she is, always has a coffee pot that's kept full in the corner. I always arrive early so I can arrange the metal folding chairs in a circle and greet the group members as they enter the room.

The diagnostic makeup of the group has changed significantly over the past four years. When I first worked as Dan's co-therapist during my internship, the patients in the group exhibited a broad array of clinical diagnoses ranging from depression and anxiety to schizophrenia and bipolar disorder with only one or two patients having post-traumatic stress disorder. However, with the massive influx of Vietnam vets over the past few years, the primary focus of the group has become PTSD.

With the addition of Richard, the Tuesday group now has

seven members: three marines and four Army veterans. All of them have post-traumatic stress from the Vietnam war. Two of the marines, Randy[3] and Butch[4], were wounded at the battle of Khe Sanh. Butch lost his left leg. Each had a tattoo on their right arm with *Khe Sanh*, the marine corps insignia, their company, and division number with the phrase *Semper Fi* under it. Two of the Army vets, George[5] and Sean[6], were in units that sustained high numbers of casualties in fire fights in the Mekong Delta and the jungles of the demilitarized zone between North and South Vietnam. The fifth member, Philip[7], was a field intelligence officer who had the grizzly task of counting dead bodies. The last member, Frank[8], who is well over six-foot tall with a muscular build and long brown hair and full beard, was an Army Ranger specializing in long-range reconnaissance patrols (LRRPs)[9] as far as the Cambodian border. Over the years, these six had all bonded over their shared stories—both horrific and heroic—as well as their physical and emotional scars.

Richard is always the last to arrive and never engages with the others in the usual preliminary greetings and chitchat.

Once everyone settles into their chairs, I announce, "Alright, let's get started," which halts the banter in the room.

Typically, when everyone comes to the circle, I wait until someone chooses to start the conversation, but tonight I have a

---

3. Name has been changed.
4. Name has been changed.
5. Name has been changed.
6. Name has been changed.
7. Name has been changed.
8. Name has been changed.
9. Long-range reconnaissance patrols (LRRPs) are specialized military operations focused on gathering intelligence deep behind enemy lines carried out by small, highly trained stealth teams whose missions involved long durations of several days or weeks.

different plan. Turning to Richard who's seated cattycornered to me, I acknowledge him directly.

"Richard, I think everyone would like to hear about your service as a marine, if you would be willing to share it."

He stares at me and doesn't respond immediately. In the silence, I can see that he's processing my request as he's never been asked to speak directly in group before. Unable to predict his reaction, the pause is making me feel anxious. *Have I made the request too soon? Is my timing right or is he not ready? Will he leave?*

Then to my great relief, he begins to talk.

"Like I told you when we first met, Doc, I joined up after high school. It was 1966, and I had just turned 18. My father was a marine, and it felt like a family tradition. I also wanted to fight the communists."

"What division were you in?" Butch asks.

"First Marine Division."

"Me, too, brother. Where were you stationed?"

Richard stares into the blank space in the middle of the circle.

"When I got into the country in '67, I was initially stationed near Da Nang, but my unit spent a lot of time north of there in the jungle.

"Growing up in Vermont I did a lot of hunting with my dad. Got to be a pretty good shot," he says, his voice going flat and emotionless. "I guess this impressed my instructors in boot camp. After basic, when they were setting up this new unit, I was asked if I wanted to be trained as a sniper. Since this felt like it would let me see a lot of action, I jumped at the opportunity."

Everyone is leaning forward. Richard has commanded everyone's attention.

"The first few months in country, my unit was involved in a

couple of skirmishes. Mostly shooting at somebody in the bush but nothing that required my skills as a sniper. That was until we got intelligence about a specific North Vietnamese unit. They had information that somebody higher up on the food chain wanted, and we were ordered to go and get it. We followed them for days until we were ready to set up an ambush at a ford in a river that we knew they'd have to use."

He pauses again and takes a deep breath.

"It was early afternoon, hot and humid. I had been sitting in the bush on a hilltop above the river ford for hours and was drenched with sweat. Suddenly, the North Vietnamese patrol emerged from the jungle and began crossing the river below me. I watched as they crossed the river. In the middle of the patrol was an officer, a colonel from the way he was dressed. More importantly, he was carrying a messenger bag over his shoulder, which I was pretty sure contained the documents we wanted. I took my time and waited until he was midway across the river and then I shot him. I saw the blood spatter from his head as he fell, and then my unit opened up from all sides until there was no one left alive in the North Vietnamese patrol. As I climbed down from the hill, I could still see his body lying in the shallow water of the ford when an intelligence officer, some CIA type, came out of the jungle to retrieve the messenger bag."

Silence fills the room. No one in the group is reacting to what has just been said, which I find odd give the graphic nature of his description. No one is making eye contact either. Everyone is staring into the collective space in the center of the circle.

Richard continues, his voice now brimming with sadness.

"I shot a lot of people in fire fights when I was in Vietnam. May have killed some. It was my job to fight those bastards, but what I did that day felt different. Oh, it was orders, and everyone was pleased at the outcome. They'd gotten the information that they'd wanted, and the captain congratulated me on a job well done. But that wasn't what I was feeling."

I can hear the emotional tensity building in his voice as he begins to speak faster.

"I couldn't get the image of that colonel out of my head. He haunted me. I kept having nightmares where I'd see him all bloody and sometimes flashbacks of him crossing the river and falling. It didn't feel like being in a battle. He wasn't shooting at me. Hell, he didn't even know I was there. It felt cold and calculated like murder. It felt wrong to me, and afterward, I knew I couldn't be a sniper anymore. When we got back to Da Nang, I transferred to a supply unit. Sometimes, even now, I just wish I had let him go."

I can feel the heaviness of his regret and the inner conflict between his humanity and the directives he was given that day. Yet, as powerful as his story is, it doesn't answer the question I contemplated on the drive down from Massachusetts earlier that evening. *Why did he attempt suicide? Did the incident with the colonel trigger it, or is there more to the story?*

As I look at Richard, I know one thing for certain: He's ready to unburden himself. In fact, he's desperate to do it.

Seizing the opportunity, I ask, "What happened next, Richard?"

Suddenly, his head snaps up, and he stares at me with that feral expression I saw in my office. I realize that I'm locked in the crosshairs of his sniper rifle.

Brushing off some lint from his pants, he tries to collect himself.

"It was the battle of Khe Sanh."

I quickly glance at the two marines who were in that battle. Both were injured there. Butch lost his leg, yet neither of them are exhibiting any external reaction despite their traumatic experience in it. They just keep staring at the space in the center of the circle.

"I had been with my new unit for a few months. We were flying supply helicopters out of Da Nang, and I was assigned as the door gunner. Our guys at Khe Sanh were surrounded and the only way to resupply them was by helicopter. We'd do a couple of runs a day. Because of the enemy mortar fire, it was too dangerous to land, so we would hover a few feet off the tarmac, and I would hand the boxes of supplies and ammo to a guy on the ground."

The emotional intensity in his voice continues to rise.

"It was the last run of the day. I was handing a box of supplies to the guy on the ground when a mortar shell exploded near us, and he was hit by shrapnel. As he was going down, I instinctively reached out to grab him. Got my arm through his flak jacket, but I didn't have the strength to pull him into the helicopter as we lifted off. I was tethered in, so I just held onto him until we got back to Da Nang. When we got there, the medics took him. He was bleeding pretty badly. I never knew what happened to him."

He pauses again, his hands bunching into fists. The muscles of his face strain with tension.

"I was rotated back to the States after that. Didn't re-up and got discharged. It was the early '70s and a bad time to be a Vietnam vet. Called us "baby killers." Lots of anti-war protests. So, I just drifted around. Traveled all over the country. Kept to myself, moving from place to place doing odd jobs. Lately though, things have changed. People seem to respect us more."

I try to bring his narrative closer to the time of his suicide attempt.

"Richard, how did you end up here at Newington?"

A glimmer of desperation flashes in his eyes.

"I heard there was going to be a Vietnam vet parade in a

town south of here, New Berlin, so I decided to go, and the strangest thing happened," he says softly. "I was standing watching the parade, all the guys were marching, some dressed in uniforms and others not, when a man comes up to me and says, 'You saved my life.' It was the guy I'd held in the helicopter coming back from Khe Sanh! He survived!"

"Amazing. You must have felt proud to have saved him," I say.

"No!" he screams as tears run down his face.

"When I looked at him, I didn't see his face! I saw the faces of all my buddies who didn't survive. They were like my family, and they were gone!" Then, in an anguished whimper, he adds, "And it wasn't just them that I saw. It was the face of the NVA[10] colonel. Just staring at me with dead eyes. Suddenly, everything came crashing back, and I had to get out of there. Got in my van and just drove around, but the visions wouldn't stop. All those dead faces and that colonel. I couldn't stand it, so I took a bunch of pills and a lot of booze. Next thing I remember, I woke up in the hospital here."

Richard falls silent, and I look around the room to assess the group's reaction, but as I search their expressions, all I see is a blankness. No one is making eye contact. No one is moving. No one is speaking. They all continue staring into the empty space.

To understand what's happening, I turn to Frank, the Army ranger who specialized in long-range reconnaissance patrols. He's sitting next to me, and we have the strongest working alliance of any of the group members because I treated him individually when I was an intern and the *Friday consultant.*

---

10. The NVA, officially known as the People's Army of Vietnam, was the military force of North Vietnam during the Vietnam war.

"Frank, everyone seems bored," I say looking at the group. "Like they're not listening to the story that Richard just told."

Taking a deep breath, Frank shakes his head.

"No, Doc. I don't know about anyone else here, but I'm not bored. I'm back in the jungle."

With Frank's comment, the other group members begin to adjust in their chairs and nod. I realize now that their reactions aren't boredom or disinterest. Each member is grappling with their own version of Richard's story.

The silence breaks and finally everyone starts talking with each other *and* with Richard. There's an emotional energy in the room that infects everyone, myself included. It doesn't feel like we're in group therapy anymore. It feels like we're sitting around a campfire deep in the jungle of war sharing the stories behind our emotional scars and the darkest thoughts we thought we'd left behind.

Months later, Richard approaches me just before group therapy begins.

"That night in group, when we all talked about what had happened to us in the war, something changed in me. I had been alone so long with my memories of that war—the flashbacks, the nightmares, and guilt, but even though we never served together, I felt a brotherhood with the other guys that I had not felt since leaving the Corps. I was no longer alone with my pain."

When Richard opened up, he began to heal, and his sense of brotherhood was restored. These are inspiring moments in therapy that sustain my motivation to do this work.

Humans are a social species and require contact with other humans to maintain a sense of psychological well-being. One of the nastier effects of trauma is that it separates people from one another, casting them into the void of social isolation and forcing them to suffer alone. However, when people come together to share their humanity, this not only repairs the broken connections but deepens them.

Sullivan observed that the therapist is not a detached or passive observer in the therapeutic process but rather an active participant-observer who's emotionally impacted and changed by the experience. Caught up in the process that night, I was not just the group's therapist but a brother of war struggling alongside them by a campfire in the middle of the jungle. While I didn't cross the boundary of sharing my own traumatic stories with them, I experienced a healing of sorts that forever weds me to their sacred brotherhood.

Questions for Consideration

1. In your opinion, what emotions do you believe the author experienced when he heard that his longtime colleague was retiring unexpectedly? What was his coping mechanism for handling his new role as a group therapist? What experiences did he have to overcome to be successful in this new role?
2. Is a participant-observer the same as a facilitator?
3. How might shared experiences, especially for veterans, assist as a coping mechanism?
4. After returning from war, do you think patients suppress their feelings or do they simply project their feelings onto someone else, perhaps whom they perceive as their next target? Do you think that the author feeling uncomfortable initially was

valid, and was his recommendation for group therapy correct?

5. Do you think that Richard was experiencing survivor's guilt? If so, do you think he felt that he should have sacrificed himself for his comrades? Could he have done something differently?

6. After coming home from war, how does one transition to the expectations of what society believes is normal? What coping mechanisms do veterans typically turn to, to dull the pain? What coping mechanisms should they try?

7. What should the military provide as a form of treatment to make sure that veterans can transition back into society in the best way possible?

8. Do you feel that the author is a true empath or just a sympathetic listener?

THE INJURED GUITARIST

---

*"If I were not a physicist, I would probably be a musician. I
often think in music. I live my daydreams in music. I see my
life in terms of music."*

— ALBERT EINSTEIN, 1929

St. Paul, Minnesota, 1989

As the Northwest Airlines Boeing 727 descends for landing at
the Minneapolis-St. Paul International Airport, the Twin Cities
emerge beyond the cloud cover. My five-year-old son, Robert,
who's been excitedly staring out the window in the seat next
to me beams with excitement.

"Daddy, look at the snow!" His reaction is quite different to
the one he had on his first airplane trip two years ago when we
were moving from West Hartford to Miami.

At that time, he was not much older than his younger

brother Richard is now, and he held on to me in fear as we landed at Miami International Airport. I tried to distract him by pointing out the window.

"Robert, look it's Miami!"

Turning to me with a quizzical look, he replied with the paradoxically concrete logic of a three-year old.

"No, Daddy, that's not *your Ami*. It's *Mommy's Ami*."

I laughed, finding the sweetness and purity of the comment amusing.

The move from West Hartford to Miami occurred when Astrid was nearing the end of her pregnancy with Richard, and I had just completed a year as the Director of Evaluation for the community mental health center in Massachusetts where I finished my residency. Focused on the needs of our growing family, we decided that we wanted our children to grow up near their grandparents and cousins, all of whom lived in Florida.

I was successfully able to secure a position as the Director of Psychology at a private psychiatric hospital nestled on the Miami River through contacts at my university in New York. Astrid, who was working as a labor attorney for the *Hartford Courant*, was able to obtain a similar position at Knight Ridder's *Miami Herald*. As we packed, I recall thinking—rather naïvely—that the future looked bright and full of opportunity.

This move felt like an idyllic fantasy, one in which I'm surrounded by warm weather under exotic palm trees playing with my children on white, sandy beaches. Suffice it to say, though, the reality of Miami in the late 1980s—the era of the cocaine cowboys—was no fantasy. Had I still been a federal investigator, there were enough schemes, scams and villains, even at the hospital that just hired me, to make a career.

After two years, it became apparent that despite the proximity of family, the social environment was not a good one for our children. So, when Astrid was offered a promotion to work as a labor attorney at the vice-president level for Knight Ridder's paper in Minnesota the *St. Paul Pioneer Press*, we jumped at the opportunity. I eventually found a position with the Level 1 trauma hospital for the area as the chief psychologist for their rehabilitation institute, and it was with a sense of relief that we boarded that 727 with our two children to leave "Miami Vice" for "Minnesota Nice".

~

St. Paul Ramsey Medical Center
St. Paul, Minnesota, 1989

It's the first day of my new position at the Medical Center and Rehabilitation Institute in St. Paul, and I keep thinking that something's off as Sheila Benson, the assistant hospital administrator who hired me, gives me a tour of the facility. I can feel a tension emanating from her that wasn't present during our previous conversations. In fact, it was her friendly demeanor and openness during the recruitment process that played a large role in my decision to take the position in the first place.

Now her voice lacks presence, suggesting that she's preoccupied with some inner conflict. It's so intense, in fact, that I'm tempted to ask her about it, but my instincts tell me that she's not ready to talk, so I refrain and try to focus on the tour.

By the time we arrive at the entrance of the Rehabilitation Institute where my office will be, she's no longer able to contain her feelings. Her voice is now quivering with emotion.

"Oh, by the way, I was let go this morning," she blurts out.

"What did you just say?" I ask, thinking I misheard her.

"I was terminated this morning. Orienting you is my last official act here. I'm sorry."

With flashbacks of my disturbing experiences in Miami, panic rises within me.

"You were let go? You're the only person I know in this place! In fact, you are the only person I know in the entire state of Minnesota!"

Noticing that she's on the edge of tears and struggling to maintain her composure, I suddenly feel the magnitude of her pain. My exasperation is not helping, so I put my hand on her shoulder to comfort her.

"Sorry. Are you okay?" I ask.

She takes a deep breath and nods.

"Dr. Gillespie, the Upper Midwest Rehabilitation Institute where you will be working has been my special project since I've been here. I recruited you because your clinical experience and training are an ideal match for what we've been developing, and you're about to meet the person who's the reason why I think that is so."

She walks me into the Rehabilitation Institute and introduces me to Dr. Rebecca

Koerner, a young physical medicine and rehabilitation physician who's the driving force behind the development of the Institute. Once the formalities of the handoff to Dr. Koerner are complete, Sheila leaves.

Becky wastes no time in welcoming me into her office and immediately starts discussing my first assignment.

"Bob, I know from your background that you have mostly worked in psychiatric settings, but here at the Institute that's not the type of patient you'll be treating. You will be dealing with similar issues of anxiety, depression, and trauma, but our patients have all sustained severe physical injuries, and, as they undergo rehabilitation, it's the psychological effects of those injuries that you'll focus on."

"So, I will be assessing and treating the psychological effects of physical injuries?" I ask.

"Yes. You'll be working on every medical unit and clinic in the hospital. The range of medical conditions you'll encounter is vast and includes everything from brain and spinal cord injuries to burns, cardiac problems, and general physical trauma from accidents including amputations."

This is a bigger job than I originally thought.

"How does my neuropsychology and psychotherapy background fit in?" I ask.

"Actually, it's ideal for the interdisciplinary treatment model I'm building here, which focuses on enhancing and restoring these patient's functional abilities and quality of life after they have sustained a physical injury or disability," she says confidently. "Your ability to do complex neuropsychological assessments and to use that information to address the issues of our patients will help guide the treatment team's efforts. It's exactly what I've been looking for."

This is music to my ears. Ever since I treated Tony, I felt this was how neuropsychology should be implemented. However, I am unsure of one thing.

"What exactly do you mean by 'interdisciplinary', Becky?" I ask.

"The Institute's staff is made up of physicians, nurses, physical, speech, occupational therapists, and social workers with each discipline having a specific role with the patient. We all work as an integrated team with our overall goal being to restore and optimize the patient's functioning."

"I see," I reply, secretly impressed by the model.

"Welcome to the team, Bob. There's a lot you are going to learn," she says, offering me her hand.

Her handshake is as firm as my old boss Charlie's. That handshake changed my life, and I can't help but feel that Becky's will do the same.

Wasting no time, Becky introduces me to the interdisciplinary team and the world of rehabilitation medicine. I find myself treating injured patients on every medical unit at the hospital except for the psychiatric ward. One of my current patients is a woman on the post-surgical unit whom the nurses are concerned is suicidal.

Arriving at the nurses' station, I introduce myself before they brief me on her condition.

"Her name is Beatrice[1]," one of the nurses begins. "She was injured in a motor vehicle accident in which four of the fingers on her right hand were severed. The surgeons were able to reattach the fingers, but the prognosis that she will regain full function in that hand is uncertain. She's a well-known classical guitarist here in the Twin Cities, and she may never be able to play again. She's been so quiet since she got here that we are worried she is depressed and possibly suicidal."

"Has she said anything that suggests she is feeling suicidal?" I ask.

"No. That's the thing. She's cooperative with treatment, but she doesn't interact with us beyond that. She just seems to sit in the bed just staring into space."

"Oh, I see. Well, let me take a look at her."

The nurses lead me to her doorway where, as they described, Beatrice is sitting up in bed staring off into space. She's a woman in her late twenties with short brown hair and

---

1. Name has been changed.

bright green eyes. Her right hand is encased in a ball of white gauze and suspended on an elevated sling.

"Good morning, Beatrice. I'm Dr. Gillespie," I say, peeping my head in the room. "I'm a psychologist here at the hospital. May I come in?"

Snapping out of her reverie, she focuses all of her attention on me.

"Of course, Doctor! Good morning!"

Crossing the room, I stand next to her bed.

"I understand you were in an accident and injured your hand?"

"Yes, terrible, terrible. Such a bother," she replies, staring at the white ball of gauze.

"Are you in any pain?"

"Oh, no. There's no pain except for the itching."

"Your fingers are itching?"

"Yes, it's the itching caused by the leeches on my fingers. It's most annoying."

"Leeches?"

"Yes, the leeches they put on my fingers."

Leeches! What kind of hospital is this?

"You think they put leeches on your fingers?" I ask, my eyes widening.

"Oh, yes. I can feel them."

Confused and alarmed, I excuse myself and return to the nurse's station.

"I think we need to get psychiatry down here for a medication evaluation. I believe this patient is having psychotic symptoms."

The nurses looked rather stunned at my request.

"What do you mean psychotic symptoms?" the nurse asks.

"The woman thinks she has leeches attached to her fingers."

The nurses look at each other and smile.

"Well, Doctor, she does."

"She has leeches on her fingers?" I ask incredulously.

The two nurses then smile at each other...again.

"Yes, Dr. Gillespie. Beatrice has leeches attached to her fingers. We frequently use leeches in certain surgical cases to facilitate blood flow."

"Leeches?" I repeat still in disbelief.

"Yes. It's quite an effective treatment. We have been doing it for some time now," she confirms. *How medieval. What's next? Bloodletting?*

A perverse image emerges in my mind as I visualize a huge auditorium filled with doctors in white coats with one on the podium proudly announcing that they will now be recommending the use of leeches after surgery.

Holding my tongue, I return to Beatrice's room to complete the consultation.

"Sorry for the break there," I say, wiping my forehead. "To be honest, I was a little freaked out by the idea of leeches."

"Oh, me too," she says, laughing. "But then the surgeon explained that it will help my healing. Strange though, don't you think?"

"Yep, but, apparently, it's very effective," I reply.

Beatrice smiles and gestures with her uninjured hand for me to take a chair near her bed.

Sitting down, I now focus on the reason for my consult.

"So, Beatrice, how are you feeling generally?"

Still smiling, she replies, "Actually, Doctor, I'm feeling fine."

"Not feeling down or anything?" I say, still uneasy about the leeches.

"No, not really. Although, I can't wait to get out of here. I have a lot of things to do," she replies, her tone pensive and low.

Sensing that she is now comfortable talking with me, I decide to explore her emotional reaction to the trauma of her injury.

"I understand that you're a classical guitarist."

"Yes," she says with a hint of nostalgia.

"Are you at all worried about not being able to play again?"

She looks at her hand with a somber expression. "Of course, Doctor."

"Feeling depressed about that?" I say, nodding toward her bandaged hand.

"No," she replies, wrinkling her brow.

Her response raises a concern that she may be hiding her true feelings. Psychological denial of injury is not uncommon in rehabilitation settings and is a complex phenomenon that has to be addressed delicately. Early acceptance in treatment can help the patient learn to adapt and remain motivated. However, if unaddressed, denial can interfere with treatment and their long-term recovery since the patient must come to a realistic understanding of any residual limitations caused by their injury.

"It would be natural to feel down about being injured like this though, Beatrice," I say, trying to assess her level of acceptance.

Suddenly, her green eyes darken, and she stares at me with fierce determination.

"I don't think you understand, Doc. I'm an artist. It's all practice and perseverance...and pain sometimes," she says, her words fading into silence. "Music for me is not just a job. It's who I am. It's the way I experience the world."

Pointing at her injured hand, she adds, "This will not change that. There is no question in my mind that I will play music again. Practice, perseverance, pain. It's how you create art. So, no, I don't feel depressed about this. I just feel determined."

Beatrice's reaction does not sound like depression or denial to me. She actually seems well-adjusted despite the trauma. Rather than denying her injury, she appears to be driven by a resolute sense of purpose, namely that with a lot of hard work and dedication, she might regain the use of her fingers and make music again.

But I can't dismiss the nurses' concerns too quickly. To them, she spaces out and stares into space for long periods of time.

"Beatrice, the nurses are concerned that when you are staring off into space, you're feeling depressed."

"Oh, Doctor! I wished they had just asked me!" she replies, taking her undamaged hand and hitting her legs. "When I'm staring like that, I am listening to the music in my head. I am mentally practicing and imaging the sound. It's like I can actually hear it and see the musical score. I can even imagine the movements on the guitar! It's like I'm playing again."

I come to realize that Beatrice is someone special—an artist. Her art has taught her a resiliency that's more powerful than any psychological treatment. As I listen to her share her love for music over the next hour, I find myself caught up in the passion that flows from her voice.

"That's wonderful, Beatrice."

"Thank you, Doctor."

After discussing my observations with the nurses, I return to the Institute and share my assessment with Becky.

"Bob, this is the type of information that's so important to know when we treat our patients," she replies, pleased with my analysis. "In rehabilitation, motivation is everything. Knowing this, the occupational and physical therapists can use it in her treatment. Sometimes this kind of information is the difference between success and failure."

I continue to visit Beatrice daily during her inpatient stay, and to my utter fascination, we continue to talk about her art. My visits change to weekly when she's discharged to outpatient care; however, the team's weekly reports are that her rehabilitation is going exceedingly well.

"The progress she's made in her finger movements is remarkable," the chief occupational therapist says in our next meeting. "I have never seen a patient work this hard. Her motivation and endurance are incredible, even when she's obviously in pain. She's practicing the exercises we give her all the time and even inventing some we didn't give her. That strange spacing out thing she does where she's experiencing music in her head seems to help keep her going. Just remarkable."

Several years after Beatrice completed her rehabilitation, I was privileged to be present when she returned to the concert stage. Her performance received a standing ovation, and was the one, I imagine, that she had been planning in her head the first day we met in the hospital.

Working with Beatrice reminded me that success in psychotherapy and rehabilitation involves not just the procedures and medications but also a complex harmony of intangible variables such as resilience, motivation, determination, and, ultimately, hope. When a patient has these qualities, it's such a positive prognostic indicator that my job is simply to find a way to reinforce their belief and make others aware of it so they can use it at the multidisciplinary level. However, when these variables are weak, or worse, the patient feels hopeless, the treatment process is compromised. To address this, therapists should establish a working alliance by joining patients on their journey, thus changing how the experience lives inside of them.

Questions for Consideration

1. How did the author feel when he found out that his recruiter was leaving her position? Why was there a heightened level of sensitivity toward someone leaving a job? Did he feel mislead?
2. What specifically did the nurses observe that indicated that Beatrice might be feeling depressed and suicidal? Why was this a misdiagnosis? Why didn't they ask Beatrice more questions?
3. Why did the author feel compelled to dig deeper into the psyche of the patient? What drove him to ask more questions about what she was feeling and thinking? What was the turning point that made him think that the nurses' assessments may have been incorrect?
4. Why did the author not want to immediately negate the nurses' observations? Being in a new position, did that change the way he approached the situation? Or did his experiences enhance the way he handled it?
5. How did the author's previous career experience help him navigate the situation with Beatrice in a professional way despite what he was feeling personally? How did he use those experiences to help his patient?
6. How did Beatrice convince the author that she was

lucid and not having a psychotic episode? How did he respond? How do you think he felt?

7. What do you think helped Beatrice more— rehabilitation or her own self-determination? Do you think that the author's trust and belief in her contributed to her success?

8. How do you think the author felt when he witnessed Beatrice perform on stage? What impact do you think that experience had on him? What impact do you think it had on her?

THE LONELY COWBOY

"Nobody ever saw a cowboy on the psychiatrist's couch."

— JOHN WAYNE

St. Paul Ramsey Medical Center
St. Paul, Minnesota, 1990

WHILE FRIDAY AFTERNOONS were always busy at the VA, at the Institute, the busiest times are Monday mornings. Requests for consultations build up because there's minimal staffing over the weekend. This particular Monday morning, I've barely arrived at my office when Becky pulls me aside.

"Bob, there appears to be a problem on the orthopedic unit. The charge nurse—who, between me and you, is, how shall I say it, a bit old school—is having problems with one of the patients. According to her, he's 'being disruptive.'"

"Being disruptive?" I ask.

"She says that he is refusing treatment and has just fired his surgeon. Knowing her, I suspect that she may be part of the issue, but, nevertheless, she's heard about your work on the other units and wants you to sort it out."

"I see."

"Also, we've been having a lot of communication and referral problems with this unit. They typically get us involved in the patient's treatment too late in their stay, and this slows down their progress. While you're up there, I'd like you to see what you can do about that as well."

Having been at the Institute for nearly a year, I feel well integrated within the team. I conduct emergency consultations and have been growing a practice with rehabilitation patients often following them from their ER admission all the way through outpatient treatment. Also, I'm doing research on the burn unit that focuses on the impact of burn wounds on interpersonal intimacy.

When I arrive on the unit, the charge nurse immediately runs toward me. Her name is Janet[1], and she's a slender woman of average height who appears to be in her mid-fifties. With graying black hair pulled into a tight bun under her nursing cap, she is dressed in a stiffly starched and immaculate nursing uniform with precise creases and a small watch pinned to her left lapel. Her rigid posture and stern, no-nonsense expression clearly conveys that she is in charge.

Foregoing social pleasantries, she points to a patient who's seated in a wheelchair staring at the unit's panoramic windows.

---

1. Name has been changed.

"It's that one with the long hair, beard, and tattoos," she says in an authoritative tone that's not used to being questioned.

The patient is a scruffy man with shaggy long hair, a scraggly beard, sleeve tattoos on both arms, and a striking neck tattoo on his left side. He's dressed in an open-back hospital gown and pants. I notice that his right leg is elevated with metal fixating rods that run from hip to ankle, giving his body a distinctly robotic look. His room is also close to the nurses' station and does not have any windows.

"His name is Frank[2]. He's a biker guy. Got injured in an accident with a truck on the interstate. Been here a month. Hasn't been cooperative since he got here," she says. "Also, he's a little too flirtatious and grabby with the nursing staff, particularly the younger ones."

I nod, remaining silent.

"And the language he uses sometimes...Well I never! But now he has gone too far. He fired Dr. Black[3], his surgeon, and that's the last straw! You can't just go and fire your doctor. Not on this unit! These patients are too ill. We can't have them firing their doctors. I will not have it! You have to do something about him. He is very disruptive."

I now know what Becky meant when she said Janet was "a bit old school." Intuitively, I feel that part of the issue is the mismatch between this nurse and the patient. However, I'm conscious of that the fact that I just received my marching orders and remain agreeable.

"Okay, Janet let me look into it."

I start by spending 30 minutes observing Frank. It's important for me to watch the way patients move as they enter the

----

2. Name has been changed.
3. Name has been changed.

therapeutic space because nonverbal information often provides significant insights into their mental state. Also, observation provides data about their pain and mobility as well as any disability they may have had before starting treatment.

As I observe the "disruptive patient," I see a man who is in his thirties sitting quietly and looking through panoramic windows. There aren't any signs of obvious agitation, but he also doesn't engage with the other patients or staff as they pass by. He only continues to sit and stare. The angle of his head, the body posture in his chair, and the lack of movement all convey a sense of poignant wistfulness.

Given that he's the subject of Janet's ire, I decide to approach him carefully, making sure to stay within his field of vision without interrupting his view of the unit's exterior windows. I speak with as little formality as possible, similar to how I might talk with friends at a bar.

"Hi, Frank. I'm Dr. Gillespie. I hear there's been a bit of difficulty and wonder if I may be of some help," I say, kneeling down beside him so we're both at eye level.

He initially avoids eye contact and continues staring out the window.

Suddenly, a deep, melodious voice speaks.

"You know, Doc, I sure would like to be out there on my own in the open country. Riding my motorcycle out past the farms, out on those prairies, and up in those mountains. Don't like being inside. Especially don't like being in that dark room they have me in."

Because of the severity of the patients' injuries on this unit, it was designed to increase efficiency by organizing the rooms in a semicircle around the nursing station, with the most severely ill patients nearest the station and the least severely ill farthest away. Unfortunately, the rooms closest to the nursing station do not have windows, but the others do.

I nod in agreement as a half-smile stretches across his face.

"But I sure do like some of these pretty girls around here," he says.

Janet was right about his flirtatious nature.

"You're not from around here, are you, Frank?"

"Hell no, Doc," he replies, turning to me. "I'm from Wyoming. Worked the ranches up that way, and if it hadn't have been for that truck skidin' sideways out there on I-35, I'd be back there now."

"You worked on ranches?"

"Yep. Pretty good life. Lots of fresh air and out in the open. Lots of freedom. Could ride my motorcycle wherever I like."

Struck by the mental image of him on a motorcycle roaring across the vast western plains, I reply, "Sounds wonderful, Frank."

His facial expression darkens. "It was 'till I got here."

My thoughts begin to whir, each one colliding into the next as the mystery around Frank becomes clearer. His issues aren't just about some deep psychological wound that turned him into the villain as Janet suggests. They're about basic human needs. He's injured and far from home. Everyone is a stranger to him. He likes wide open spaces and doesn't like to be cooped up inside. The flirting with the nurses? That's about feeling lonely.

However, there's an edge of hopelessness in Frank's eyes. The change in his voice conveys more than just frustration at being in a facility. He's holding onto a deeper emotional pain that's yet to be explored.

"Frank, are you feeling anxious?" I ask.

He turns his head away from the windows toward me.

"Doc, if you were sitting in this chair with this leg,

wouldn't you be?" he says, his voice constrained with a fear that he can barely control.

With this leg...

I look at his leg. It's held together by metal from top to bottom. This is a surgical technique used only for the most complex bone fractures when the risk of losing the limb is high.

"Frank, why did you fire your doctor?"

"Why'd I fire him? Why'd I fire him? Look! Look!" he yells, pointing to a group of patients standing by the windows. They're all on crutches, each with a leg missing. "He's their doctor, and I'd like to keep both my legs!"

Click. Another piece of the puzzle falls into place. Frank is terrified he's going to lose his leg, and, with it, his independent lifestyle of working on ranches and riding his motorcycle. Exacerbated by having to depend on strangers, these fears have triggered a survival response in the most primitive part of his brain. Feeling helpless and vulnerable, Frank has done the only thing he can do to restore control over his life—resist the team's treatment efforts and attack the nucleus of his fear and distrust by firing his surgeon, Dr. Black.

With this realization, I start to develop a plan of action, but I still need a bit more information about what has happened between him and the nursing staff.

"Well, I guess I can see your reasoning on that, but what about the nurses? They're just here trying to do their jobs and help you."

He nods his head toward the nursing station where Janet has been intensely observing our conversation.

"Some of them are all right," he says, "especially the younger ones. They are easy to talk with unless that old one, who's in charge, is around. They're all afraid of her, and she don't like me. She don't like the way I look or how I talk. She especially don't like me now that I fired that doctor. She and him are pretty tight, and neither one likes me acting independently, so, when she's here, they avoid me. In this place everybody's got to follow her orders."

The final piece of the puzzle drops. Frank's problem isn't with the nurses. It's with Janet, and, based on my brief conversation with her, I have to agree with his observation. Her rigidity has intensified his feelings of isolation—something alien to his freewheeling lifestyle.

Sorting out this mess will require not only joining him in his struggle but doing so in a manner that does not heighten the conflict between him and Janet.

"I believe you got that right about the nursing staff, Frank," I say, pausing to let my words sink in. "You know, Frank, I'm not from around here either."

"Yeah, I heard that in your voice, Doc. I know you ain't from out West where I come from either. I'll bet you're from back East. Maybe New York?" he says suddenly smiling.

"You got me, Frank. Grew up in New York City," I reply, concocting a new plan. "So, what do you say? Let's us two outsiders fix up what's been going on around here—between you and the nurses."

"What do you have in mind, Doc?"

My assessment of Frank differs from Janet's. Rather than being an obstreperous, crude, discourteous individual, he seems to possess a sharp acumen for social observation and interaction. The behaviors that she's upset about are caused by the fear of losing his leg and the resulting social isolation, but they don't reflect the totality of the man. At his core, his self-image is that of a cowboy, able to roam free and live independently.

His self-concept is also attached to a romantic ideal of courtly, courteous behavior toward women, which has been temporarily lost in this moment of crisis. However, his quaint phrase *These pretty girls around here* gives me the hook I need to unravel his problematic interactions with the female nurses. I need to help him reconnect with this side of himself as it might not only calm things down with Janet and the staff, but it may also reduce his feelings of helplessness.

When dealing with patients who feel alienated, I will sometimes use a mirroring technique drawn from the ideas of neurolinguistic programming (NLP)[4]. For example, I may subtly change my style of speech and cadence to match theirs or adopt a similar physical posture to theirs when communicating with them. It's similar to a *call and response*[5] in singing or music. Done well, the patient unconsciously identifies with the therapist and joins in the therapeutic enterprise. So, as I make a proposal to Frank, I shift to a more colloquial style of speech.

"I don't know how it works where you come from, but where I come from, if a guy wants to court the ladies, he acts gentlemanly. You know, all courteous and polite with 'pleases', 'thank-you's' and 'yes ma'ams' and 'no ma'ams'. And not much cussing either. Think you can do that?"

I guess I haven't been the easiest guy to get along with these last couple of weeks. I'm just so worried about this damn leg, but I'd be willing to try and be more courteous, if they will," Frank admits, smiling.

"You do your part and let me work on them for you, okay?"

---

4. Neurolinguistic programming (NLP) is an approach developed in the 1970s by two psychologists, Richard Bandler and John Grinder, that focuses on how one communicates with themselves and others and how this influences their behaviors and behavioral outcomes.

5. A form of interaction between a speaker and one or more listeners, in which every utterance of the speaker elicits a verbal or nonverbal response from the listener or listeners. In music it refers to a style of singing in which a melody sung by one singer is responded to or echoed by one or more singers.

"Sure, Doc. I'll give it a try."

With the alliance between us tentatively established, place my hand son his shoulder. "And looking good wouldn't hurt either. How about if I arrange for one of those pretty young nurses to help trim your hair and beard?"

"Don't think I'd object to that. Not at all," Frank replies looking up at me with a mischievous grin on his face.

"Also, if it's okay by you, I'd like to keep meeting with you to see how our plan is going."

"I'd like that, Doc. You're really easy to talk to—even if you are from New York."

A smile flashes across my face.

"Oh, and one last thought, Frank. If you're getting worked up about your leg, I want you to stare out those windows. See the mountains and see yourself riding your motorcycle through them. It also wouldn't hurt to take a couple of slow deep breaths while you're doing it."

"I like that idea, Doc."

My therapeutic alliance with Frank is the most important tool in my arsenal, and I need him to know that I'm going to act on his behalf to execute our plan. I'm also aware that my performance is being intensely scrutinized by the nursing staff and Janet, so it's time for some stagecraft.

Standing up, I return to the nursing station to confer with Janet. She's standing slightly outside the edge of the station— the boundary of her domain—as I nod to beckon her over.

"Well, Doctor, what is your assessment?" she asks, standing with her arms crossed.

Positioning myself so that Frank has a clear view of me, I sharpen my gaze to appear stern and serious.

"He's frightened about losing his leg, and this is a strange place for him."

"But what about firing Dr. Black?" she replies, ignoring what I just said.

This gives me an opportunity to accomplish Becky's second mission about involving the Institute earlier in patient treatment.

"Oh. I can't help you with that. Frank doesn't trust him, and there is no fixing that. You and the medical staff will have to figure that out, but I suggest that you talk with Dr. Koerner, who might be able to help since she will eventually be in charge of his rehabilitation."

Having planted the idea, I return to my plan to help Frank.

"I think I can get him to behave better," I continue. "He will be taught relaxation and coping strategies to help him deal with his fear. We'll also be working on his social skills. Once he's more comfortable with me, I will arrange for a psychiatric consult since he's going to need some medication to help buffer his stress but not yet. He's too distrustful."

Brows slightly lifted, Janet is intrigued by my suggestion.

"What I need for you and the nursing staff to do is to remember that underneath his bravado and gruffness, he is frightened about losing his leg and to take that into account when you deal with him," I say, leaning closer and softening my tone. "Think of what it would feel like to be in that wheelchair with all that metal attached to your leg."

Janet gives me a steely look. Empathy is apparently not her strong suit, so I return to my more authoritative doctor-nurse demeanor and give her a direct order.

"I would like him moved as soon as possible to a room with a window. He is used to being out in the open. This will improve things and will aid in his recovery. I will also be on this unit seeing him every day."

"You'll see him every day?" she asks suspiciously.

"Yep."

Janet's face softens, and I make my final pitch.

"Janet, I would also like you to do me a favor and have one of the younger nurses offer to trim his hair and beard."

Her arms and shoulders stiffen. "You'll be on this unit every day?" she repeats.

"Yes."

"And you'll arrange for psychiatry to do the medication consult?"

"Yes."

She pauses, contemplating her next move. "Will you talk to Dr. Koerner about taking over the case?"

I smile knowing that Janet has taken the bait. In her mind, this is her pound of flesh in exchange for the haircut deal, but in reality, this is just what Becky wanted me to arrange in the first place.

"I'd be glad to do it, and I'm sure I can get her to agree."

"Okay. I'll see what I can arrange about the haircut."

I look over at Frank and give him a quick conspiratorial nod and wink. He smiles in return. I leave the unit and return to the Institute to confer with Becky, who's pleased with the outcome. What I don't know, however, is whether Frank's agreement to the plan will last.

When I return to the unit the next morning, the situation is noticeably different. Frank, who is looking quite coifed with a neatly trimmed haircut and beard, is busy having a lively conversation with a young nurse. He's also sitting in front of one of the rooms with a window.

 Not wanting to interrupt them, I stop by the nursing station to speak with Janet. Her body language is more relaxed. She even smiles at me.

"It's been a better day today," she says, dryly. "We were able to move him last night to a room with a window and, since then, he's been more cooperative with my staff. In fact, the nurse who cut his hair said that he was quite courteous and even funny with her when she was doing it. Not at all rude. Also, Dr. Koerner called to say she would agree to take him as one of her patients."

"That's great," I say. "Thanks for your help. I put in for the psychiatry consult, which will happen next week, and I'll continue working with Frank to keep things stable."

Janet nods, and I approach Frank who's just finished his conversation with the nurse. As he looks through the windows, I pull up a chair beside him where we can both soak in the landscape.

"You know, Frank, I love the high desert country of the southwest, and when I look out those windows that's what I see."

"Not me, Doc. I just see the mountains and plains of Wyoming."

"Either way, Frank, it's a beautiful and peaceful image."

"You got that right. And Doc?"

"Yes, Frank?"

"Thank you."

"It's my pleasure, Frank. Now tell me a bit about yourself. Where did you grow up in Wyoming?"

With this question, Frank's psychotherapy begins. I see him every day while he's on the surgical unit, and once a week during his months of outpatient rehabilitation with Dr. Koerner at the Institute. We focus on his motivation for treatment and the adjustments to his lifestyle due to his injury.

Despite his reservations about his surgeon, Frank's leg eventually heals. Once the metal fixators are removed, the physical therapists help him regain full strength and mobility in his injured leg. At times, this is a painful process, but Frank exhibits remarkable determination. After 12 months of intense treatment, he's finally able to resume normal ambulation.

Frank also continues to be gentlemanly with the nurses, and he becomes one the physical therapy staff's favorite patients—so much so that on the day of his discharge, all of the staff except Janet gather at the main entrance to the hospital to bid him farewell.

A few of his biker friends wait outside for him with his motorcycle, which they had arranged to have repaired after his accident.

Walking through the doors of the medical center on two good legs, he mounts his motorcycle, starts the engine and revs it to the sound of freedom and the open road. He then turns to the assembled staff, and with a wave of his hand, he gives us a courteous bow. Everyone spontaneously claps for him as he roars down the highway with his biker friends.

Of course, Frank being Frank, he doesn't put on a helmet, which makes me worry about his safety, but as he disappears into the sunset, I start to miss him. Frank didn't just charm the nurses and the physical therapists; he also charmed me.

The core issue in Frank's psychotherapy, and what was driving the behaviors that Janet labeled as "disruptive" was his fear of not just losing his leg but the freedom that came with it. As I worked with him and other rehabilitation patients, I came to realize that physical injuries, much like psychological traumas, not only damage the body but also damage one's sense of self. Once I was exposed to this fundamental truth on a daily basis, I realized that in working with patients like Billy, Manny, Elena, and Tony, and Frank, one must remain close to the patient's journey to truly help them heal. The role of the psychotherapist is first to help them reactivate their sense of psychological well-being, as this is the foundation underlying the human capacity for compassion, purpose, and resilience. It's not enough to simply restore a patient's physical functioning or alleviate a specific symptom; they must be equipped with the understanding, awareness, and knowledge that they, too, matter.

Questions for Consideration:

1. Did Janet stereotype Frank as being disruptive and unruly because of how he looked and spoke before she knew what was truly going on with him? How do you believe she assessed him? How does this differ from the author's assessment of the patient and the people that were treating him?

2. What was Frank's goal in reacting to the surgeon and nurses the way he did?

3. Why do you think the author's compassion and empathy for the patient caused him to open up and go along with the plan? Was the patient already open and just in need of someone to bring out his personality? Why did this "cowboy" trust the author who was from New York?

4. How did the author's observation of the patient assist in his success in getting him to open up? After the author's assessment, how did he adapt his communication style to relate to the patient physically and culturally? Would the author have been as successful if he hadn't been willing to change or adapt to the patient's needs?

5. Do you think the author's treatment of Beatrice influenced the advice that he gave to Frank? If so, how?

6. What traits or characteristics did the patient exhibit that challenged the nurses, physical therapists, and the author?

7. What did the landscape enhance and/or inhibit Frank's treatment and healing?

8. Why do you think that Janet didn't come to Frank's farewell send-off? Do you believe she was dug into her own assessment of who he was that she couldn't see that he had the ability to change and be the "ideal patient"? Why is control to some people more important than the actual treatment of the individual? Would you want this person overseeing you or your treatment?

THE ANGRY GIANT: BETHESDA—PART 1

"From the ashes, a fire shall be woken, A light from the shadows shall spring..."

— J.R.R. TOLKIEN, 1991

St. Paul Ramsey Medical Center
St. Paul, Minnesota, 1991

IT'S EARLY MONDAY MORNING, and I am finishing my second year at the Institute. I've just driven into the office from my home in North Oaks, a picturesque suburban community situated on a nature reserve near Pleasant Lake just outside of St. Paul. The soft summer air smells sweet, and the countryside is lush with greenery after the harsh Minnesota winter. The outpatient rehabilitation clinic, which is not open for another hour, is quiet and peaceful.

As I sit at my desk preparing for my rounds, the phone rings.

"Dr. Gillespie," I answer, holding the phone to my ear with my shoulder.

"Good morning, Dr. Gillespie. It's Sheila Benson."

"Sheila Benson!" I shout, grabbing the phone. "How the heck are you?"

I haven't heard from her since she gave me the tour on her last day of work at the medical center.

She explains that she's now the administrator of Bethesda Lutheran Memorial, a rehabilitation hospital that's a few blocks away from the medical center and the Institute. But I sense that she's not just calling to update me on her career shift.

"Dr Gillespie, I would like your help with a problem at our hospital. We are using an outside psychologist, and I don't think the quality of his services is very good. Worse yet, we are losing money, which is not happening with any of the other clinical services we provide. We can't figure out why this is happening and since you are doing similar work, I'm wondering if you can take a look and make some recommendations."

Sheila has always been kind to me. Remembering the tears in her eyes when she was let go, I agree to meet with her the following week to examine their files—a task that's eerily reminiscent of my days as an investigator.

Lutheran Rehabilitation Hospital
St. Paul, Minnesota 1991

Early Monday morning, I meet with Sheila at the rehabilitation hospital. We tour the facility and its various programs before I start examining the spreadsheets of their psychology services. We agree to meet at the end of the day to discuss my findings.

"So, what did you find?" Sheila asks anxiously.

I spread the financial statements across the table.

"Sheila, the problem is that you've outsourced your psychology services," I say, lifting one of the documents. "And you're not billing for them like you bill for your other clinical services. You're actually paying way too much, and I think that if you build your own in-house service and bill for it in the same way as you do for your physical, occupational, and speech therapy services then you will stop losing money and begin to make a profit."

Sheila purses her lips as she contemplates the idea.

"Actually, you should consider expanding what you are offering," I continue. "Given the scope of your current inpatient rehabilitation programs, my analysis indicates that there are significant unmet clinical needs for psychological and neuropsychological services and if the hospital bills them correctly, this could increase your overall revenues," I say, pointing to one of the spreadsheets.

Sheila nods but remains silent. I thank her for giving me the opportunity to help her and return to the Institute.

A week later, I receive another phone call from Sheila.

"Bob, could you come over to the hospital to have lunch with me and Dr. Ormiston, our medical director? He would like to discuss your recommendations about psychology and neuropsychology services here at the hospital. I think you'll like him. He's been the driving force behind developing most of the programs here."

Over sandwiches, she introduces me to the hospital's medical director, Dr. Charles Ormiston. A tall man with thinning brown hair, he exudes an infectious folksy charm, which makes me like him instantly.

As we eat, he explains that he's a neurologist by training and that, in addition to being the hospital's medical director, he runs its stroke rehabilitation program. He also shared that, like me, he is not a native Minnesotan.

"Sheila told me that you're originally from New York City. Well, I grew up in Four Corners, North Dakota, which was aptly named since if you stood in the middle of Main Street, you could see all four corners of the town. My great grandfather walked there from Pennsylvania in the 1870s to open a lumber mill."

I smile and nod.

"Dr. Gillespie, it was me who asked for the review of the psychology services. I was dissatisfied with the quality and scope of what was being provided and was taking heat from administration over the costs. I knew that there was a problem, and your analysis has been quite enlightening."

Pleased that he's happy with my findings, I graciously thank him for the opportunity. But I also have a gut feeling that we're not here just to talk about paperwork.

"Dr. Gillespie, Sheila and I have been talking to the higher-ups here at Bethesda, and we want you to hire you as our psychologist," he says, not mincing any words.

"Thank you, Dr. Ormiston. I'm flattered that you want to hire me, but I must respectfully decline," I say, humbled by the offer. "As I told Sheila, there is simply too much work to be done at your hospital for one individual psychologist. Given the range of rehabilitation programs you're running, you are going to need to build an entire psychology-neuropsychology service, and this would require hiring several psychologists and neuropsychologists, not just one. Also, I have to be very honest, I am quite happy at the Rehabilitation Institute. Dr. Koerner is teaching me a lot, and I get to do research. So, I must decline the offer."

Sheila sinks into her chair and folds her arms.

"Well, think it over, Dr. Gillespie. I know that I am going to."

As we pack up the rest of our sandwiches, I politely thank them for the offer once more and return to my office at the Institute.

The next morning, Sheila calls again.

"Dr. Gillespie," I answer.

"Dr. Ormiston wants me to set up a meeting with you, him, and some higher-ups at the hospital," she says disregarding all social pleasantry.

"What is this about, Sheila? I thought I made it clear that I didn't want the job."

"Bob, I don't really know, but he has been closeted with the hospital's president, the CFO, and the HR Director all morning, so I expect it's something bigger than just discussing hiring you as our psychologist. Also, no lunch this time. The meeting is in the administrative conference room, and I have not been invited. So apparently, it's above my pay grade."

Intrigued but dubious, I agree to the meeting. Sheila and I meet at noon at the rehabilitation hospital's entrance, and she escorts me to the conference room in the administrative suite.

"I have Dr. Gillespie," she says as she shuts the door behind her.

The conference room is dominated by a long rosewood conference table surrounded by high-backed leather executive chairs, four of which are occupied. Dr. Ormiston, who is wearing his white lab coat with a stethoscope around his neck welcomes me in, as three unfamiliar administrators watch me carefully. The two men are wearing gray business suits and appear to be in their early forties. Dr. Ormiston introduces them as the hospital's president and its CFO. The woman, who's perhaps in her mid-fifties and dressed in a gray pants suit, is the director of human resources.

As we settle around the conference table, Dr. Ormiston's demeanor is relaxed and friendly. The others remain stern and serious, causing me to feel a bit uncomfortable.

"Dr. Gillespie, after reviewing your analysis with Dr. Ormiston, we are convinced that you are correct and that the hospital needs to expand its psychology and neuropsychology services," the president of the hospital begins. "My CFO also informs me that your idea to create an in-house service will solve our financial problems. In short, we are inclined to agree with your proposal to build an in-house psychology-neuropsychology service and would like you to come here and build it for us."

My proposal? Had I proposed that I build this service for them?

When I agreed to the meeting, I suspected that there would be a counteroffer to take the psychologist position (probably involving more financial compensation), but I didn't anticipate them agreeing to implement my suggestions since it would require a significant investment.

Momentarily flustered, I tug at the collar on my shirt and decide to wing a reply.

"You realize that since you'd be starting from scratch, I would have to recruit a team, which takes time, and the financial problems wouldn't get straightened out until you were sufficiently staffed and could provide enough services to meet your patients' needs, right?"

The hospital president smiles for the first time in the meeting, nodding first to the HR director.

"That is why she is here. She will help you hire your staff, and that should speed up the recruitment process," he says, now nodding toward the CFO. "And that's why he is here. He will work with you on the billing problems."

And that's why this guy is the president of this place...a very clever fellow indeed.

Looking across the table, I see Dr. Ormiston smiling.

"This is a big project and a very big ask," I reply. "I'd like to think it over."

Throwing a questioning glance at Dr. Ormiston, the president says, "Fair enough. You're right. This is a big project. However, Dr. Ormiston thinks it's a necessary one for us to grow, and I agree with him. So, take some time and let Sheila know what your decision is."

As we depart the meeting, Dr. Ormiston escorts me toward the door and pauses, holding on to the door handle.

"Bob, I know you like it at the Institute. Becky Koerner is a great doctor, and I think she has done an excellent job mentoring you with respect to the medical rehabilitation model, but I believe you and I can build something unique here."

"I'll think about it, Dr. Ormiston."

This time I'm a lot less certain about my answer.

The offer and Dr. Ormiston's comments trigger a week of obsessive agonizing and repeated late-night discussions with Astrid—all of which culminate late Sunday afternoon with me sitting in my car at the top of the parking ramp at Bethesda. From where I'm parked, I can see both hospitals: Bethesda looming above me and, in the distance the medical center where the Institute is housed. I again weigh the pros and cons of the offer.

My current position at the Institute represents security—a safe haven where I feel established but with limited potential for growth. Bethesda, on the other hand, represents an opportunity to create a cutting-edge program that could be a vehicle to explore more ideas about neuropsychology, psychotherapy, and rehabilitation.

With my car quietly idling in the waning afternoon sunlight, it suddenly becomes clear to me that I did not leave my position with the government and my roots in New York City just to come all this way and play it safe. I have the opportunity to build an entire clinical department from the ground up. With this realization, my anxiety evaporates, and I drive home to tell Astrid about my decision.

Early the next morning, I call Sheila to accept the position and meet with the HR director. However, I delay staring my new role at Bethesda for a month so that I can wrap up my clinical work at the Institute and say a goodbye to Becky Koerner and the staff who've taught me so much about rehabilitation.

As I'm packing up my office, Becky stops in to say goodbye. A look of somber recognition fills her gaze.

"Bob, I'm sorry to see you leave. You did good work here. You learned our treatment model quickly and everybody liked you and respected the work you did, but I think we all knew you weren't going to be here long term. You seem to be seeking something. I think you're a bit of a dreamer."

"Maybe so, Becky," I reply.

"Well, to do the job you're taking on at Bethesda, you'd have to be. That place is growing by leaps and bounds, and I don't think anyone knows what it will look like in the next few years. I'm glad you'll be working with Charlie Ormiston, though."

"Why is that?"

"I've known Charlie for a long time. He's an excellent neurologist, but, more importantly, for what you two are cooking up, he's a dreamer too. You're kind of oddly well matched."

Becky's assessment proves accurate. Over the next few years, Dr. Ormiston and I form a powerful working alliance and, eventually, a friendship that allows us to not only build the psychology and neuropsychology department we envisioned but also manage a clinical crisis that was created in response to an unusual offer from the State of Minnesota.

Bethesda Lutheran Rehabilitation Hospital
St. Paul, Minnesota, 1994

It feels surreal that three years have passed since I was offered a position to build and direct the hospital's psychology and neuropsychology service. Walking into the administrative conference room with the rosewood table and high-backed executive chairs where I was once interviewed, I see Dr. Ormiston, the hospital's president, CFO, HR director, Sheila, and the directors of nursing, physical, speech, occupational therapy, and social work.

We've been summoned to meet with a special representative of the governor of Minnesota, a pleasant and soft-spoken woman named Marsha[1]. After being introduced by the hospital's president as a registered nurse on the governor's staff, she

---

1. Name has been changed.

explains that her job is to identify unmet medical needs in the state and to develop programs that address them. I watch her carefully as she pulls out a thick binder from her briefcase.

"The state of Minnesota would like Bethesda to create an inpatient treatment program for patients with brain injuries who have histories of violence. The goal of this program will be to rehabilitate and reintegrate them back into the community," she begins.

A bit skeptical, I lean back in my chair. *This is a naïve idea since there's no cure for brain injury. If patients have become violent as a result of their injury, then there's no cure for the violence. Also, treating violent patients will present significant risk to our staff and other patients.*

Looking around the table at the other clinical department heads, I see similar doubtful expressions. That is, except for the Director of Nursing who nods repeatedly about the idea.

"Why would the state fund such a project?" the president asks.

Marsha opens her binder and thumbs through her notes.

"Several years ago, there was a lawsuit in the state of Texas brought by the family of a young man who had sustained a severe brain injury and became violent."

In Texas, as everywhere else, some individuals who sustain brain injuries exhibit chronically violent behavior. These individuals typically require institutional care in facilities that have the capacity to manage and subdue them when they become aggressive. Since almost all patients with this level of injury eventually end up on Medicaid—the state funded insurance—this means that tax dollars are spent on their care. At the time of the lawsuit, Texas did not have such a facility and had to outsource this type of treatment to programs in other states, specifically a program at Worcester State Hospital in Massachusetts. This meant that Texas patients were sent out of state to a place far from their families and that Texas taxpayers paid for it.

Marsha explains that the family of the young man were upset at not being able to visit their son and brought a suit against the state arguing that Texas tax dollars should not be spent this way and that the state needed to develop its own program. When the family won their suit, the state of Texas was not only forced to develop a program, but it lost a great deal of money and suffered tremendous embarrassment.

"There is a similar situation with a family here in Minnesota. Their son suffered a brain injury in a motor vehicle accident and has become very violent. He's now at the same treatment facility in Worcester, Massachusetts as the patient from Texas. Since everything is being paid for by our Medicaid dollars, they are threatening to bring the same lawsuit against the state of Minnesota that succeeded in Texas. To avoid such costly litigation, the governor has decided to develop an in-state program, which is why we've come to you."

I breathe a sigh of relief. At least the proposal is not a naïve act of beneficence but rather a pragmatic solution to a costly legal problem. However, it still doesn't make it any more feasible to accomplish.

"Marsha, such a program, if it could be created, is likely to have a long length of stay for its patients. Even for rehabilitation hospitals like ours, which by design have a much longer average lengths of stay than traditional hospitals, the average stay is still only about 30 days. Doubling or tripling that to 60 days or 90 days still doesn't give us enough time to accomplish what you're proposing," I say.

Marsha smiles like the cat that ate the canary. Leaning forward in her chair and placing both arms confidently on the conference table, she says, "That's an excellent point, Doctor.

With respect to length of stay, we are prepared to pay for up to two years of inpatient treatment for each patient."

That response causes quite a stir in the room. The hospital president and CFO who are seated at the end of the table are now wide-eyed with excitement due to the financial impact this will have. I can tell they're already sold.

I clear my throat, deciding to voice my own concern.

"My second question is about outcome. Even if we are successful in figuring out how to control the violence on an inpatient unit, where would these patients go after discharge? Patients with this level of neurological impairment are unlikely to be able to live on their own."

Marsha leans back in her chair with the same air of confidence she had during my first question.

"Ah, yes. The discharge question," she says. "Once you've rehabilitated these patients, we anticipate that they will be discharged to specialized group homes[2]. We've already been working with several companies to develop them and expect

---

2. *Group home* commonly refers to a residential environment in which a small number of unrelated people in need of care, support, or supervision due to mental or physical disabilities live together. The development of community-based group homes for individuals with brain injuries had an interesting history. Initial efforts to place individuals with brain injuries in group homes designed for the mentally ill proved unsuccessful because individuals with brain injuries did not have the same behavioral dynamics and characteristics as those with chronic mental illness, which led to dramatic behavioral disruptions including conflict with the staff and other residents. Similar attempts to place them with individuals with developmental disabilities also failed for the same reasons. Specifically, individuals with developmental disabilities were working to achieve a higher level of functioning that they had not yet achieved, while individuals with brain injuries were trying to recover the level that they had lost. Ultimately, it became clear that mixing diagnostically different clinical populations within group homes was not a good idea and that the specific needs of individuals with brain injuries required the development of specialized group homes.

them to be available when your first patients are ready for discharge."

No one has any more questions and the hospital president, who's still goggle-eyed, ends the meeting stating that he will review the proposal and remain in touch.

Two weeks later, we return to the same conference room for another meeting with the hospital president, CFO, HR, and Sheila. This time Marsha is not present. However, I notice someone new seated at the table.

The hospital president announces that he has agreed to the deal with the state and that we will build a new unit to develop the program. It's going to be called the Neurobehavioral Brain Injury Program (NBI). The Director of Nursing introduces the man across from me as the NBI program manager who will be in charge of design and implementation.

John[3] is a tall lanky man in his late twenties with long black hair pulled into a ponytail. He's dressed in a white lab coat, and I make a mental note from her introduction that he's both a nurse and a colleague of hers from a prior hospital.

Looking around the table at each of us, he says, "It will be a high-tech and highly secure unit with bulletproof glass windows and doors with electronic locks. The unit will be built in a circle with ten patient rooms. There will be an in-unit conference room, two treatment rooms, a padded quiet room, and a nursing station, all of which will be enclosed by bullet-proof glass. In the middle of the unit, there will be a common area. All the furniture, tables, and chairs will be bolted to the floor. The patient rooms, however, will have Dutch doors to

---

3. Name has been changed.

facilitate communication with them while they are in their rooms."

It occurs to me that the Dutch doors don't match the high-security design of the rest of the unit, but I keep that thought to myself.

As he continues, we learn that the unit is going to be run by nurses who will organize the day-to-day programming and manage the patients. The various clinical departments will provide specialty services, including physical, speech, and occupational therapy as well as social work services. My department is going to be in charge of providing neuropsychological assessments. Dr. Ormiston will be the medical director for the program alongside an appointed physiatrist[4].

My main concerns are about the physical risks to the unit's staff who will be interacting in close quarters with these patients. It's unclear how we're going to control their violent behavior, and my doubts intensify when the neuropsychology staff, who have experience working with brain-injured patients, are relegated to the relatively minor role of conducting neuropsychological assessments and will not be actively involved in treating the unit's patients. This will be done by the nursing staff.

After the meeting, I voice my concerns to Dr. Ormiston, but he simply shrugs his shoulders in frustration.

"Bob, there's hospital politics and money involved," he says.

*Politics and money...*Suppressed memories of my government investigations come flooding back.

"The reason they selected Bethesda is that the Director of Nursing is close friends with Marsha," he continues. "They

---

4. A physiatrist is a medical doctor who specializes in physical medicine and rehabilitation.

went to nursing school together at the U. So did John, and they convinced the hospital's administration to let nursing to run the show. Heck, I'm the medical director, and I don't feel in control. There is a lot of emphasis on getting this up and running but not much discussion of the treatment model they will be using. It all seems a bit rushed to me, but there isn't much you or I can do about it at this point. We'll have to just wait and see."

I brush my hand against my lips. At least my staff will have limited exposure to potential physical risks, but I feel sorry for Dr. Ormiston who's titularly in charge of this circus.

Despite the complexity of building a hospital unit with high-level security, the construction is completed in a month, and the first patient is admitted within two weeks. It appears that the nursing staff are managing the unit well, and, after a month, there are five patients on the unit and no injuries to the staff or reported incidents of violence from the patients. However, everything changes when a patient from a psychiatric unit in northern Minnesota near the town of Hibbing is admitted.

The patient, Tom[5], is a huge man. Standing six feet, six inches tall, he is built like a football linebacker. According to his medical records, he sustained a cerebral aneurysm in his right frontal lobe[6], which has made him so uncontrollably violent that he requires continuous hospitalization and sedation. Seeing him during the admission process raises my anxi-

---

5. Name has been changed.
6. A burst cerebral aneurysm in the right frontal lobe refers to the rupture of an abnormal bulge in a blood vessel located in the frontal lobe of the brain.

ety. *He is a giant and will be quite the handful to manage if he gets agitated.*

This is in direct contrast to the concerns of his family members who accompanied him from their family farm located near International Falls along the Canadian border. They collectively emphasize the importance of making sure that he brushes his teeth and seem unconcerned about both his belligerent behavior and the potential risks for injury that he presents for our staff.

During the drive home, I can't shake the ominous feeling in the pit of my stomach. Astrid and I spend time making dinner and conversing about our day, but by the time we go to bed, I'm still wired and can't sleep.

When I finally begin to drift off, the phone next to our bed rings. I squeeze my eyelids before glancing at the clock. *It's 1:00 AM.* Groggy, I pick up the phone and a sobbing voice of a nurse startles me awake.

"Dr. Gillespie! There's been an incident on the brain injury unit! The police are here! Dr. Ormiston says he needs you STAT! The place is a wreck! You have to come in! Please come quick!"

"I'm on my way!" I say, hanging up the phone. "There's been an emergency at the hospital, and I have to go in," I say to Astrid.

"Go. I will take care of the boys."

Keying myself onto the unit, I'm shocked by the chaos and destruction that has taken place. It looks like a bomb exploded. The chairs and tables that were once bolted down are now scattered all over the unit. The bulletproof case that surrounded the nursing station is nothing more than thousands of glass shards strewn about the room.

Some of the nurses are too shocked to talk and others are sobbing. Two burly St. Paul police officers stand by the door while the nurses sit on what's left of the chairs. Dr. Ormiston,

John, and Sheila huddle together in the center of the unit. All of them have anxious expressions on their faces. As I approach, Dr. Ormiston breaks away from the others and pulls me aside.

Pointing to a young, petite nurse who's weeping uncontrollably, he says, "I want you to help her. She was almost killed and is in bad shape emotionally. I've given her a sedative. However, before you do that, talk with the night charge nurse, Mary[7]. She can fill you in about what happened here tonight."

"On it," I reply still trying to process the destruction.

"Bob, this is not good," he adds cryptically. "Not good at all! There are a lot of problems here."

I nod and walk over to Mary who's talking with the other nurses. We have a good working relationship, and when she sees me approaching, we find two unbroken chairs and sit down to talk privately.

"My God, Mary! What the hell happened?" I ask.

She fights back tears, trying to compose herself.

"Dr. Gillespie, I don't know how this could have happened. I think it's just that this program and all our staff are so new."

I nod as she recounts the events of the night. The meaning of Dr. Ormiston's cryptic comment becomes clearer when I learn that there'd been a catastrophic systems failure both on the unit and in the hospital. Memories of Mike and Lilly briefly cross my mind.

The event began with a communications failure during the shift report between the evening and overnight staff. This is a transitional procedure that takes place at the change of shift and involves the nurses on the earlier shift reviewing the status of each patient and discussing their needs with the

---

7. Name has been changed.

incoming staff. The nursing station on NBI is designed with a room in the back for this purpose.

"From what I can piece together, Dr. Gillespie, for some reason, the nurse who was assigned to Tom for the afternoon-evening shift didn't give him his medication and also didn't inform the nurse assigned to him at shift change," she says as another wave of emotion hits her.

"About an hour into our shift, when we were trying to get the patients back into their rooms to get ready for bed, Tom started becoming agitated and wouldn't stay in his room. When we tried to lock him in, he just climbed over that damn Dutch door and started roaming around the unit. We couldn't redirect him. He just wouldn't listen, and the more we tried to control him, the more agitated he became. Eventually, his agitation escalated, and he just started bellowing incoherently. I could see that the situation was getting out of control and told the other nurses to get the other patients, who were confused and frightened, locked in their rooms. We then retreated to the nursing station and called the patient assistance code over the hospital intercom."

Mary begins to sob. I put my hand on her shoulder to comfort her, but she continues to whimper.

"Nothing happened. No one responded. No one came to help," she says, taking a deep breath. "I saw him through the window in the nursing station. Wandering around. Bellowing like some crazed beast, and then he started ripping out the chairs and tables that were bolted to the floor and throwing them around. We tried calling the code again, but still no one came."

"No one came?" I ask incredulously.

Mary begins to sob even more.

"It was like we didn't exist. We were trapped in the nursing station with this mad man between us and the unit's only exit. For a moment, none of us could think of what to do."

Mary now points to the petite woman sitting at the nursing station weeping, her voice choked with emotion. "That was when Jenny[8] came back onto the unit from her lunch break, and everything went from crazy to dangerous."

Her complexion turns pale and she starts to shake. Clearly overwhelmed, she stops talking and I rub her shoulder waiting for her to regain control.

"When Jenny keyed herself back on to unit, she, like everyone else in the hospital, had no idea that we had called a code. She couldn't have been on the unit for more than a few seconds when Tom targeted her. He ran over and, towering over her, picked her up and began carrying her around like she was a toy doll. She started kicking and yelling but couldn't get away."

I look over at Jenny who's sitting with two other nurses. She's crying and has a distant stare in her eyes.

"We thought he was going to kill her, so we all rushed out of the nursing station and created a distraction, jumping, yelling, and waving our hands. Thankfully, it worked. Tom was momentarily distracted, and Jenny was able to get loose. Once she got free, we all ran back to the nurses' station. That's when all hell broke loose."

All hell broke loose? How could it have gotten any worse?

"After Jenny got away, Tom got even more enraged, but now he was focused on us. He picked up a chair he had ripped out of the floor and started banging it against the bulletproof glass window that was between us and him."

Mary takes a deep breath. I reach and hold her hand.

"You must have been terrified."

---

8. Name has been changed.

"It was horrible! He just kept banging and banging on the glass, and the noise was deafening...and then...," she says, starting to take short, ragged gasps, "the glass came loose from its fittings and shattered, exploding into the room. There was nothing between him and us. Nothing! And then he started moving toward us through the empty window space, roaring like some prehistoric beast."

A later examination of the issues on the unit revealed that there was a design flaw in the construction of the bulletproof window of the nursing station. It was not the correct type of glass and had been incorrectly anchored into the window frame.

Mary tugs on her uniform, taking a few deep breaths to calm herself.

"We were trapped and completely exposed, so we all retreated back to the report room at the back of the nursing station. It was the only place to go."

This space is a windowless conference room used for shift change. It only has one door for entry and exit, but it does have a telephone.

"Once we were all in the room, we couldn't see Tom anymore, but we could hear him tearing up the station and throwing the filing cabinets and furniture around. Then, he started pounding on the door. It didn't have a lock, and two of us had to lean against it as he tried to force it open. You could see the door moving as he pushed against it. It was then that I came to my senses and dialed 911. It took half an hour for the police to get there, and all that time he was trying to get at us."

I meet with Dr. Ormiston later that night, and he explains that the police entered the unit with their guns drawn. Tom didn't attack them, but he stopped bellowing and walked out of the nurse's station, stepping over the Dutch door, and sat down on his bed.

"Bob, I think he recognized their blue uniforms as some type of authority symbol, and it calmed him. Very strange."

I decide that it's best not to reply, because, as a psychotherapist, Tom's reaction isn't strange. It's human development and learning. We all learn as children the significance of a policeman's uniform and, even in his primitive state of rage, Tom's neocortex remembered it and reacted accordingly.

We decide that in the future all personnel will wear either white lab coats with the hospital's logo or scrubs so that the patients will recognize them as staff members who are there to help them. It proves to be an effective strategy.

After finishing my conversation with Mary, my immediate job is to provide emotional support to the traumatized nurses, especially Jenny, who's frozen expression hasn't changed from the moment I saw her. She's eventually referred to the hospital's Employee Assistance Program[9] and requires psychological treatment for post-traumatic stress disorder. She never returns to either to NBI or the hospital.

As the morning sun starts to rise, I debrief with Dr. Ormiston and Sheila and finally return home exhausted.

I manage to snag a few hours of sleep before returning to the hospital the next day, but as soon as I arrive to my office, the phone rings. It's Sheila and she wants to meet, but when I arrive at her office, she's not alone. Dr. Ormiston is with her and is the first to speak.

"Bob, later today we are going to begin a full hospital-wide

---

9. An Employee Assistance Program (EAP) is a voluntary, work-based program that offers free and confidential assessments, short-term counseling, referrals, and follow-up services to employees who have personal and/or work-related problems.

debriefing of what happened last night. It's going to involve the Director of Nursing, the entire NBI nursing staff, all department heads, and anyone who has worked on NBI as well as the HR director."

I nod attentively, knowing that something huge is about to be unleashed.

"Bob, this whole NBI project has been botched from the get-go, and it's time to make some changes. The root cause of what happened last night is that they rushed this whole project and cut corners. The construction was shoddy, and they didn't do nearly enough training of the NBI staff or the hospital as a whole. The staff here are highly trained to deal with the problems of physical rehabilitation and medical crises like code red for cardiac emergencies or the other codes for weather and fire disasters, but they were not trained on how to respond to the psychiatric patient assistance code that was called last night. That's why the hospital staff who were on last night were not sure what the code meant or what they should do. So, they did nothing."

Deciding that it's time to be frank, I look Dr. Ormiston directly in the eyes and say what I've been thinking since the first meeting with Marsha.

"You and I both know it's more than that. The real root causes of what happened last night are greed and power. The project was rushed from the beginning because the hospital's administrators saw a financial windfall, and the nursing department made a power grab. If those dynamics are still at play, what's going to change?"

Expecting Dr. Ormiston to challenge my blunt analysis, I brace myself for his rebuttal.

"Bob, you're right, which is why I met with the hospital's president and HR director this morning. I told them that I was going to resign as the medical director of NBI if they didn't fix the problems on the unit. They have been totally embarrassed by this disaster and are worried about the liability for what happened to the nurses on the unit and about how the hospital's board of directors may respond. So, they agreed to my terms."

"Your terms?" I ask.

"Well, first, they have agreed to hire a national consultant who specializes in building this type of unit to look at the construction flaws and how to fix them. In their rush, they hired local guys who had no experience with this type of high-security unit. It'll cost them money, but I think they now recognize the real risks and liabilities involved. I also made it clear that I wouldn't be involved if they didn't do it right."

"So, they are just going to fix the physical problems on the unit and nothing else?" I reply still distrustful of the hospital's administration.

"Oh, no! That's just the beginning. There is going to be a change in the leadership of NBI. I think after what happened last night that it's pretty clear that it's not working out with the program being under nursing."

"What happened to John, the unit's program manager?"

"He resigned early this morning."

I feel terrible for John. While this wasn't an ideal situation, I enjoyed working with him.

"And this is where you come in, Bob. I want you to assume the responsibility of directing NBI," Dr. Ormiston continues. "This will be in addition to running your department. Everybody working on that unit will report to you and I want you to mold them into an interdisciplinary team, similar to the approach you learned at the Institute."

I'm stunned by what he has just proposed, but I have to consider the risks involved. A dramatic change in leadership is needed, but getting everyone to cooperate is an organizational nightmare given the politics of the different departments. I know Dr. Ormiston isn't making this request lightly. Suddenly, I'm more concerned about my own fate than John's.

Sensing my hesitancy, Dr. Ormiston's facial expression softens.

"Bob, you and I have worked well together for the past few years. We've successfully expanded the role of psychology and neuropsychology in every program at this hospital and have begun to change the way the staff here approach rehabilitation. We have an opportunity to achieve something extraordinary for a clinical population that everyone has given up on. If you can organize and manage the staff, then I have some innovative treatment ideas that might change things for these patients. So, what do you say?"

It's the moment of truth. Am I in or out?

There are risks to what he's proposing, but there are always risks. There were risks to accepting his offer to leave the Institute just like there were risks to leaving all I had in New York for an internship at Newington a decade before. Risks will always be a fundamental part of life, but this proposal is about more than weighing the risks. It's about my belief in our clinical partnership, and, ultimately, trust—something that he's earned by supporting me as we implemented our shared vision for the hospital. This is the same trust that I felt with Charlie Annibale as a field agent. It's the knowledge that come what may, he would have my back. It's the kind of trust that allowed me to take the necessary risks in the field to complete an investigation. It's the kind of trust that resolves my doubts and allows me to take on a project that's ripe with clinical risk.

"Let's do it," I say, getting up from my seat and extending my hand.

Dr. Ormiston stands up and gives me a firm shake, clasping my left arm with his other hand.

"Yeah! Let's do it!" he says, the anger in his voice replaced with resolute determination.

Questions for Consideration

1. Was there an element of fear or dismissiveness from "the powers that be" because the administrators saw a money grab? Did that play a bigger role than the hospital's expertise leading up to this disaster?
2. Do you think that the author should have spoken up? If he had, would that have meant career suicide?
3. Why do you think that the staff were not properly trained on the missed code? This was before cellphones, so why do you think that wasn't addressed beforehand? Who do you think should be held accountable for this situation? Who do you think was the mastermind behind it?
4. What reservations did the author have when he accepted the offer of Dr. Ormiston? What does it take to have implicit trust with someone with their life and career on the line?
5. Do you think a month was enough time to put together a facility of this magnitude and train the staff properly? Were there proper protocols set in place during shift change to make sure everyone knew what was going on?

THE TRAPPED SOUL:
BETHESDA—PART 2

"The meaning of life is to help others find the meaning of theirs."

— VIKTOR FRANKL

Bethesda Lutheran Rehabilitation Hospital
St. Paul, Minnesota, 1994

IN THE AFTERMATH of Tom's rampage, the first step is to repair the unit and correct the design flaws. As agreed upon by the hospital administration, they bring in a national consultant to oversee the project. New bulletproof glass is installed and anchored correctly not just for the nurse's station but throughout the unit. The Dutch doors are replaced with solid doors with small windows that serve as view ports to observe the patients without entering the room. Also, the "quiet room" is redesigned to meet clinical standards with high-tech material that cannot be scraped off the walls and eaten. More importantly, Sheila takes on the responsibility of training the hospital staff to respond to patient assistance codes and implements several other safety protocols with input from the nurses.

Clinical services offered to patients are offered on a minimal basis during construction, but the hiatus proves to be a golden opportunity for me and Dr. Ormiston. We meet with the staff along with the other departments to discuss the change in leadership and the new structure of the program. To my relief, there's no resistance, and everyone, including the nursing staff, is enthusiastic about the changes. This may be due to the trauma everyone is feeling, though.

The major organizational change I make is to create two interdisciplinary treatment teams similar to the ones I worked on at the Institute under Dr. Koerner. Led by a neuropsychologist, each team consists of a speech, occupational, and physical therapist as well as a social worker and a nurse. Out of an abundance of caution, I assign myself to lead one of the teams.

The neuropsychologist will coordinate patient care and their individualized treatment plans based on the collaborative input of each member of the team whose focus is to identify the triggers for the patient's violent episodes. From there, we devise medication, behavioral, and environmental regimens to reduce the frequency of these episodes with the hope of eliminating them altogether.

Initially, I insist that no patient can be admitted who I have not personally assessed. However, as my confidence in the interdisciplinary teams' operations increases and NBI's patient census[1] grows, I eventually relinquish this responsibility to the other team leads. Fortunately, everything goes well, and we don't have another Tom incident.

Anoka Regional Treatment Center
Anoka, Minnesota, 1995

Six months into NBI's reorganization, I make the trip to southeastern Minnesota to evaluate a man hospitalized at the Anoka Regional Treatment Center (formerly Anoka State Hospital). He's been referred by a social worker from the facility who describes him as non-ambulatory[2], mute, and violent.

Anoka is the fourth state hospital created in Minnesota for psychiatric patients deemed to be "incurable." Originally opened in 1900, it was also the first state hospital in Minnesota to be designed according to a cottage plan—a progressive treatment concept that housed faculty and patients in individual buildings organized in a campus-like setting around a central green space. The purpose was to reduce the institutional feel of the facility and provide more specialized treatment for patients by organizing them into groups with similar diagnoses.

As I enter the facility, it feels anything but warm and

---

1. Patient census refers to the count of patients receiving care on a given unit in a healthcare facility at a specific time and is crucial metric that impacts staffing and resource allocation.
2. A "non-ambulatory" patient is unable to move or walk independently without assistance. In Sonny's case, while he could pull himself about on the floor independently, he was unable to sit-up, stand, or walk freely. Much to the nursing staff's dismay, he could punch and bite though.

inviting—an impression that's not dispelled by the hospital's administrator, a dour and overweight man in his fifties. Balding with a fringe of brown hair, he's dressed in a rumpled blue business suit and gives me the distinct impression that I'm wasting his valuable time.

His eyes narrow when I explain my willingness to evaluate, let alone consider admitting, this patient.

"That's all well and good, Doctor. I'm sure your program is excellent, but I really doubt if it's going to be able to fix this one. He's been here a year, and I haven't seen any change in him. Even though he can't walk, he is so strong that he can rip a radiator out of a wall while prone on the floor. He has punched and bitten our staff so hard that when we try to do his daily cares[3], we have to keep him restrained and heavily sedated most of the time. Also, he likes to smear his feces."

Quite pleased with his description of the patient, he dismisses me with a wave of his hand.

"But, if you still want to take a look at him, be my guest. I have more important things to attend to. I'll have one of the nurses take you to him."

A few minutes later, a nurse in a white uniform leads me to a room in the back ward of one of the hospital buildings. The room is bare except for a bed where an African American man in his mid-thirties lies in restraints.

According to the hospital records, he was admitted the prior year after having been badly beaten in a mugging in Chicago. During the attack, he was thrown down a flight of concrete stairs and fractured his skull, causing severe brain damage.

------

3. "Daily cares" for a non-ambulatory patient refers to taking their vital signs, administering medications, performing required hygiene, feeding them meals, and noting any changes in their patient's condition.

Even though he didn't sustain a spinal cord injury and has full use of his arms and legs, he's unable to stand or walk independently and can only sit up with assistance. According to nursing records, he mostly pulls himself around on the floor. He can, however, punch, kick, and bite, and he has injured several of the hospital's nurses, behavioral techs, and patients. The nurse tells me that he's incredibly strong and has torn apart beds and ripped radiators and other equipment off the walls. She also confirms that he smears his feces.

His chart states that he's mute and has not spoken coherently since his admission to the hospital. He's also had frequent nightmares during which he yells and screams.

The patient's name is Raymond[4], but everyone calls him Sonny. According to one of the social workers who interviewed his sister on the telephone, it's apparently a nickname that he acquired before he was injured because he looked like the heavyweight boxing champion, Sonny Liston, who fought and lost his championship in the 1960s to Cassius Clay—before Clay became Muhammad Ali.

No family has ever come to visit him at Anoka and, unfortunately, because of his violent episodes, most of the hospital staff are afraid and avoid him. Consequently, he's been socially isolated since his admission.

As I observe him strapped down in the bed, straining to lift his arms and moving his head from side to side, he appears to be quite muscular despite not having the ability to exercise or walk. When I comment on this, the nurse speculates that pushing against the restraints and pulling himself around on

---

4. Name has been changed.

the floor are like doing isometric exercises[5], which may account for his muscle tone.

Despite feeling apprehensive, I sit down next to him on the bed.

"Sonny?" I say as he continues to yank on the restraints. "I'm Dr. Gillespie, and I'd like to help you."

Suddenly, he stops straining and his eyes lock on mine. He's mute, but there's something that I see (or maybe just feel) about the look in his eyes. It conveys a sense of desperation, like there's intelligence trapped inside of a body unable to free itself. That expression combined with what I now know about the history of his injury and his treatment at Anoka solidifies my decision. *I'm not leaving him here.*

"Tell the hospital administrator that I'll take him," I say, turning to the nurse.

"Really? You're sure?" she replies in disbelief.

"Yes. Our admissions people will help set up the transfer and transportation."

Shaking her head, she turns and walks away, leaving me to find my own way out.

As I exit the facility, I feel a twinge of doubt and wonder how I'm going to explain this decision to Dr. Ormiston and the NBI staff. The long ride back to St. Paul doesn't help, but as I recall the look in Sonny's eyes from his hospital, I feel more confident I've made the right decision.

Unfortunately, Sonny proves to be quite the handful after he's admitted to NBI. The nurses decide that it's safer for him to sleep on a mattress on the floor due to his risk of falling out of bed, and, oddly, he seems to like this arrangement. He also engages in the same aggressive behaviors—punching, biting,

---

5. Isometric exercises are exercises that involve the contraction of muscles without any movement in the surrounding joints.

kicking staff, and destroying things much to the hospital administration's disapproval and my waning popularity. Fortunately, though, he hasn't smeared feces on the walls, but if and when he does, I fear there will be an all-out insurrection amongst the staff.

~

Bethesda Lutheran Rehabilitation Hospital
St. Paul, Minnesota, 1995

Thanks to the reorganization of the NBI and the new safety protocols, Dr. Ormiston is able to test a theory he has about violent, brain-injured patients.

"Bob, I think that these patients have been so violent from the onset of their injuries that they have been overmedicated with psychotropics[6], especially sedating ones, since being injured," he says over coffee. "I believe that these medicines, especially at the dosages they were given, have interfered with their brains following the normal neurological recovery progression and are contributing to their problems."

I nod in agreement. "Yes, the excessive use of sedating medications is certainly consistent with the clinical histories we have for these patients."

"Bob, I want to briefly take the patients, even Tom, off all psychotropic medications."

My heart rate speeds up as my body tenses at the memory of Tom's rampage.

Ignoring my reaction, Dr. Ormiston continues, "I want to

---

6. Psychotropic medications are drugs that act on the central nervous system to alter brain function, helping to regulate mood, cognition, and behavior.

take them to ground zero[7] and then reintroduce the psychotropic medications one at a time to observe their effects."

"That's a risky proposal, Charlie. Think about what happened when they missed Tom's medication. Also, it's going to be a tough sell to the nursing staff who have the primary responsibility for managing any outbursts."

"Yes. I've thought about that," he says undeterred. "I recognize that, for a time, the episodes of violence are likely to increase, but since the reconstruction and reorganization, NBI is a different program. The unit is more physically secure, and the staff are better trained in how to manage violent incidents, and the hospital-wide training Sheila has been doing with the patient assistance codes means we have plenty of back-up. Also, this will be a planned medical intervention, not an unexpected random event, and I believe any risk will be rapidly mitigated."

Unconvinced, I take another sip of coffee.

"Not only have these patients been overdosed with psychotropic medications, but I believe that injured brains do not respond normally to even standard doses of these types of medications, so when I reintroduce them, I'm going to use micro-doses instead of the standard or mega doses."

"Micro-doses?" I ask.

"Yes, I'm going to use the lowest dosages of these medications available and may even cut those in half. We'll only introduce additional medication when needed so we can measure their effects. If I'm right, we'll start to see them follow the expectable recovery pattern from their brain injuries."

"Taking everyone to ground zero and then micro-dosing

---

7. Ground zero: Slang for the starting point or the most basic condition or level.

them. Charlie, that is a heck of a proposal," I say, feeling nervous, cup still in hand.

∼

Dr. Ormiston's idea of microdosing is revolutionary, especially with this clinical population. The dominant model for prescribing psychotropic medications has always been "more is better" with most psychiatrists applying *macro*-dosing to their patients, especially those that don't respond to the standard prescription amount.

However, because the staff trusts him, or rather, because I trust him, I hesitantly agree to test his theory. One at a time, we take each of the patients off all their psychotropics and then introduce microdoses of nonsedating and mood-stabilizing medications.

The patients, including Tom, respond better to the microdoses. While it doesn't completely eliminate their violent episodes, their frequency and intensity decline dramatically. Better yet, they become more predictable.

Once this occurs, the treatment teams are better able to identify the environmental and behavioral triggers for their episodes and develop behavioral strategies to either manage them or avoid them all together. Soon, the patients become ready for discharge to the group homes that are being prepared in the community.

While it takes time to make the appropriate medication adjustments and identify the triggers, it doesn't take as long as I had anticipated. As we learn more about what microdoses are most effective for each patient and the teams become more experienced with identifying behavioral triggers, the average length of stay for the patients is about 90 days, which is nowhere near the two years that Marsha from the governor's office had generously offered to authorize during our initial meeting.

Unfortunately, though, while the other patients, including Tom, improve, Sonny's case proves to be more difficult. He continues to lash out and bite the nursing staff during his daily cares, and his treatment team is unable to control his violent outbursts. Everyone is growing increasingly frustrated, discouraged, and negative toward Sonny, which is making me question my decision to admit him.

I know that the staff is at a tipping point. It's been six weeks since I admitted him, and I can hear the murmurs echoing down the corridors.

"Gillespie made a mistake admitting him."

"He put us all at risk. What was he thinking?"

"Even our program couldn't help this patient! He should be sent back to the state hospital."

"Ormiston can't fix this one. His ideas are crazy. Maybe he just got lucky with the others."

We are definitely running out of time with Sonny.

Around 8:00 PM on Saturday night, I finally make it home to relax with Astrid. As we discuss the day's events while the boys play, the phone suddenly rings. Grabbing the receiver, I hear the night-charge nurse's voice on the line.

"Dr. Gillespie, you have to come in!" she says excitedly.

My mind immediately jumps to Tom's rampage and my heart races with anxiety. All I can imagine are crying nurses, broken glass, and overturned furniture.

"Has there been an incident? Are the police there?" I ask, gripping the phone tightly with both hands.

"No, No. It's not like that," she replies. "It's a miracle!

Sonny is sitting in the common area talking to one of the nurses. He even remembered his sister's phone number in Chicago. We called it and he talked with her! Please come and see! It's a miracle!"

Astrid looks at me with concern in her eyes. She also lived through the Tom incident and knew how much it had upset me.

"Is it the hospital? Has there been another incident?" she asks.

"No, honey. It's the opposite. I think we've had a breakthrough with one of our most difficult patients. I have to go into the hospital."

"Go. Go. Call me when you know more," she says, relieved.

After kissing the boys on their heads, I give Astrid a hug and race to the hospital.

When I enter the unit, my eyes can't believe what they're seeing. All the nurses are gathered around a table in the common area where Sonny is sitting and joking with them. Everyone is smiling and laughing.

I sit next to Sonny at the table, making sure not to disrupt the cheerful atmosphere.

"Hi, Sonny, do you remember me?" I ask.

"Sure do, Doc. You brought me here from that other hospital."

We speak for about 15 minutes, and he's remarkably lucid. He's able to remember several details from both his hospitalization at Anoka and at the NBI. He does not, however, remember being injured, which is common for traumatic brain injuries.

He shares with us what he remembers about his stay at Anoka. As he speaks, my mind recalls the look of desperation I saw on his face—the embodiment of trapped intelligence seeking a way out.

"Doc, there is a lot about being there that I don't remember. It's all very foggy. I remember feeling frightened because I couldn't get my body to work right. I wanted to stand, but I couldn't. There are flashes of people coming and going and moving me around and touching me. I remember not liking it. I hated it when they strapped me down and remember being angry at them but not being able to tell them. It was like being trapped in a dark cave that I couldn't get out of. It was horrible."

He then looks intensely into my eyes with the same expression I saw the day I met him at Anoka.

"Then you came, and you said you wanted to help me. I remember when our eyes locked. I wanted to scream so badly 'Yes, help me please!' but I couldn't. Yet, somehow, I knew you understood me even without the words."

"Yes, I remember that moment quite vividly, Sonny. I'm not sure how I understood you, but I did. It was like more of a feeling, but I knew for certain that you wanted our help."

We both pause to relive the emotion of the moment.

"Sonny, tell me what happened today."

"Doc, it was like my mind and body suddenly woke up from a long sleep. My head was clear, and I was able to move again and, best of all, I was able to speak."

"They tell me you remembered your sister's phone number and that you talked with her?"

"Yes. I haven't seen her in years. I grew up in Chicago but moved away a long time ago. You know, Doc, before I got hurt, I was studying in New York at the Culinary Institute of America to be a chef. My sister told me that when I got hurt, I was about to graduate and had come back to Chicago to invite everybody from the family to my graduation. I'll have to take her word about being in Chicago, though, because I don't remember much about it."

After 15 minutes, Sonny's eyes begin to droop, and I can see his energy fading.

"Sonny, you've had a long day, and I suggest you get some rest. We can continue our conversation tomorrow. I'm going to have the nurses change your room to one with a normal hospital bed if that's okay with you."

"I'd like that very much, Doc," he says, smiling.

Once everything is prepared, he slowly leaves the table. He's slumped over, and his legs appear stiff, but I watch in amazement as the man who once dragged himself around on the floor and smeared his feces on the wall now walks to his room with the assistance of two nurses, completely lucid.

Excited, I call Dr. Ormiston.

"Charlie, this proves your theories about microdosing psychotropics and the negative effects of overmedication for this type of patient!"

"Bob, this is just the beginning," he says, clearly pleased about Sonny's progress. "I think there's a lot more to learn about what we are doing. We are going to have to carefully study this treatment approach and duplicate it with a lot more patients before I'll be certain of how reliable it is. But, for now, we've had a big win. Also, I don't think the staff will want to fire us anymore, at least not for a while."

We hang up, but just before leaving the unit, I pull Mary the charge nurse aside.

"Quite different from the night when Tom went on his rampage, isn't it?"

"My God, Dr. Gillespie, you and Dr. Ormiston have pulled it off!"

～

The excitement about Sonny's recovery starts to wear off as, he slowly starts to regress. In a week's time, he has stopped walking and become mute again. While he hasn't resumed his aggressive outbursts during daily cares, I can see that the entire staff are worried about him and are experiencing a crisis of confidence in our treatment approach once again.

Fortunately, Dr. Ormiston remains remarkably calm, as if he expected this, and slightly increases the microdose of Sonny's medication. Within 24 hours, Sonny is able to walk and communicate with the staff again and never regresses during the rest of his stay at NBI. Another miracle.

On Friday, we review Sonny's progress in his office. Dr. Ormiston looks at Sonny's chart with a focused gaze.

"Bob, I'm thinking that the microdose approach may have to be individualized for each patient. The specific medication and dosage that works for Sonny may not work for Tom or another patient. Like I said, there is still a lot of work to be done to perfect this model."

This proves to be true with the wide range of patients admitted to NBI over the next few years. The core idea is to avoid overmedicating them and use microdosing so that they can follow the normal neurological healing progression. This allows us to personalize their medications and microdoses to their individual needs. While human brains all have a similar neuroanatomy[8], no two brains function exactly alike, and no two brain injuries cause precisely the same symptoms.

Because of the physical and neurocognitive deficits Sonny

---

8. Neuroanatomy refers to the physical structure and organization of the brain and nervous system.

suffered, he required about six more months of inpatient rehabilitation before he was ready for discharge to a group home. The day he was scheduled to leave the hospital, I met with him to discuss his discharge plans. His attitude toward living in a group home and reintegrating into society was positive, but there was one thing left on his mind that he wanted to discuss.

"Doc, you know before I got injured, I was studying to be a chef," he says. "I know I'll never be that now. Can't remember new things too well. Sometimes, I wonder if it would have been better if I had died. If I hadn't come here, I would still be at that other hospital and that's not a life anybody should have."

This discussion shakes me. Sonny, who was strapped down in a bed at Anoka, is now having a philosophical conversation with me about the ethics of treatment.

As we talk, I recall the look of trapped intelligence that I saw in his eyes that day. *What would have happened to him if I had missed it, and what was it that triggered what I experienced?* I'm startled by the thought that, even with all my clinical training, in some ways, I still operate like a field agent in the streets using my intuition to organize minimal data into a fact pattern I can act on.

The impact of Sonny's awakening as a result of Dr. Ormiston's hypothesis and high-risk decision about microdosing had a profound impact on the NBI staff. It changed how we viewed future patients who were lost, locked in a cage of their own suffering, but who, with our help, would eventually be able to return to their community and have a semblance of a normal life. During the remainder of the time that I was the Director of NBI, no one who had been working in the program when Sonny woke up ever left and the near revolt due to my and Dr. Ormiston's judgment transformed into a deep and abiding commitment to the NBI project.

I have come to think that one doesn't leave the place where they witnessed a miracle. Experiencing an event like Sonny's changes a person. It can make them believe in something higher than themselves and stay to be a part of it. As a brilliant speech therapy colleague of mine, Trisha Nance—who, years later, worked with me to create a brain injury foundation in St. Louis—once put it: "Bob, we brain injury treatment folks are kind of like a cult. We're believers, and once you get in, you never leave."

For me, directing the NBI program at Bethesda was perhaps the most significant experience of my professional career. It completed the transformation in my clinical thinking about the application of neuropsychology and neuroscience to the treatment of clinical conditions—a transformation that had begun years earlier in the lonely experimental laboratory at the University of Connecticut's Alcohol Research Center and had been shaped by my experiences at Newington and the Institute. Looking back, it has always felt to me like a mystical time, when the stars aligned to create something unique and positive in the world.

A year after Sonny woke up, I returned to the Anoka State Hospital to evaluate another patient for admission and met with the same dour hospital administrator who had dismissed Sonny as a lost cause.

After I completed the evaluation of the patient, he pulled me aside.

"What ever happened to that guy you took? You know the one who couldn't walk or talk and was so aggressive that we had to restrain him all the time? Bet you had to discharge him to another state hospital, right?" he asked smugly.

"Well, no. He's actually living in a group home in Edina and has a job making pizzas at Pizza Hut," I reply with a politeness bordering on correction. "Did you know he wanted to be a chef before he got injured? Even studied at the famous Culinary Institute of America in New York. He turned out to be one of our most successful patients."

The administrator's jaw drops and his eyes widened in disbelief. He tries to form a coherent response, but no words escape from his lips.

Questions for Consideration

1. How did the NBI retain people after the "Tom incident"? How was that incident instrumental to getting things changed to run their own program and make their own decisions?
2. How did the author and Dr. Ormiston handle the situation as leaders and calm people down to get them onboard with the program? How did they make them feel secure? Did they offer mental health services?
3. What did they do to make the trainings more effective for the staff so that people would feel safe? How did they make safety a priority for the employees in such a complex and complicated situation where people could be seriously injured or killed?
4. What legal components would have come up after Tom's incident, especially involving the nurse that didn't come back? Do you think that there were compensation or services offered to her to help her to move on from the situation?

5. How did Dr. Ormiston come to the conclusion that micro-dosing was the answer for Sonny and the other brain-injured patients? What do you think made him realize that patients were being overmedicated? Why didn't the author buy into his idea right away? Was it because of the patients' violent tendencies or was it something else?

6. When the author met Sonny, he states that he had a gut feeling about him. How do feelings factor into science?

7. How did the emotion and attitude of the staff change when Sonny woke up and became coherent? How did the staff's confidence level rise because of these successes? Why was there zero turn over? Why were the staff so committed? Would you be that committed after an event like that?

8. Why was the first option in these types of situations to overmedicate and what made Dr. Ormiston come to the realization that maybe introducing micro-dosages was better for the brain and its healing?

9. How do you think this situation impacted the author's wife, Astrid, who had "lived" the Tom situation in her own way? How was her support instrumental to a complex and complicated situation that called the author away from his family on an ongoing basis, especially knowing that they were sometimes violent and dangerous?

10. Why was the director at Anoka so dismissive of the patient? Why was the only option for this administrator to give him medication and restrain Sonny? Why do you think that the patient was

referred to the NBI? Was it because they wanted to get rid of him and make it someone else's problem or that they wanted to prove themselves right that he could not be helped?

11. When the author came back to evaluate another patient, why was the hospital administrator so shocked that the author and his team were successful in helping Sonny? Why wasn't he willing to learn from that experience to make his program better?

THE DEVOTED DAUGHTER

"The golden rule: An underlying medical illness or medication side effect has to be ruled out before ever deciding that someone's symptoms are caused by mental disorder."

— ALLEN FRANCES, M.D. *2012*

I-94 East
Between St. Paul and Milwaukee, 1999

THE BLACK LINE of the interstate stretches out in front of me toward the horizon. It's a moonlit winter's night, and on both sides of the road, farm fields are buried in snow, reflecting the endless glow of glistening stars. The temperature outside the cab of my Bronco II is below zero. Occasionally, I put my hand against the driver's side window to feel the cold against my skin.

Driving east on I-94 from St. Paul, I head toward my home and family in Mequon, Wisconsin. It's a route that I've become familiar with over the past 18 months ever since Astrid's career took her to the *Milwaukee Journal Sentinel.* I've been commuting to Bethesda and the NBI ever since, but tonight's journey is different.

My eldest son, Robert, has fallen ill. His symptoms are baffling the doctors in Milwaukee, and I have come to the realization that the long commute is no longer possible. I'm leaving Bethesda, a place of miracles, in search of my own.

There is no doubt regarding my decision to leave. My primary focus has to be on Robert and his recovery, but as I drive east through the dark wilderness of the snow-covered countryside, another emotion consumes me. Perhaps it's a combination of grief at leaving Bethesda, the NBI, and Charlie behind as well as uncertainty about my future.

The long drive helps me to realize that my decision to leave Bethesda is simply the next step in a professional journey, which has been a clinical odyssey of sorts—one that has pulled me from my roots in New York City to New England, then to Miami and back north to Minnesota and now to eastern Wisconsin (or the "Heartland" as my Midwesterner friends like to call it).

As I stare through the car's windshield at the dark horizon ahead, I'm comforted by the thought that come what may, my journey is not a solitary one. Buffering my uncertainties are the images of Astrid—my partner, collaborator, and trusted consigliere—and my two sons, Robert and Richard. While there may not be a road map for the journey I'm on, they are my north star reminding me that I'm a husband and a father first and a clinician second.

~

Pain Management and Treatment Center
Mequon, Wisconsin, 2000

While my son receives treatment, I decide to delve into a few clinical projects to keep from worrying myself to death. One of these involves working as a neuropsychology and rehabilitation consultant to a small rural hospital just outside of Milwaukee. There, I meet a woman named Dr. Pamela Thomas-King, an anesthesiologist fresh out of a medical fellowship at Duke University.

Over lunch in the hospital's cafeteria, she tells me that she's opening a freestanding clinic for pain management. Listening to her speak reignites my interest in the psychological effects of pain, especially chronic pain[1], and the strategies I've learned at the Institute and Bethesda to help patients.

What especially attracts me to Dr. King's treatment approach to pain management is its comprehensive interdisciplinary nature[2] that focuses on improving the patient's overall functioning, not just medicating their pain. This multilayered approach is similar to the methodology used at the Institute and with Dr. Ormiston at Bethesda. Given this alignment, I agree to become the psychological consultant to her clinic.

---

1. *Chronic pain* is pain that persists for longer than three months and may continue even after the initial injury has healed or may not have a clear cause and is distinguished from *acute pain*, which is short term (lasting less than three months), has a specific cause such as injury, surgery, or illness, and usually resolves once the underlying cause is treated.

2. Comprehensive pain management strategies refer to a holistic approach to treating chronic pain that considers the patient's overall well-being and integrates various clinical interventions that address physical, emotional, and psychological effects of pain on a patient's life.

Dr. King and I sit in her office during my second week to discuss a patient that she is particularly concerned about.

"Bob, I consider Julia[3] to be a high-risk patient, and I am going to need your help to treat her effectively," she says, thumbing through a thick medical file folder.

"Why do you consider her high risk?" I ask.

She pulls an X-ray out of the file and holds it up to the light.

"She has severe chronic pain from degenerative disc disease that has not been relieved by multiple back surgeries and a spinal fusion[4]. She also has a history of multiple suicide attempts with several psychiatric hospitalizations. Given the nature of her back problems, there is only so much that I'm going to be able to do for her medically. My concern is that her pain may trigger a severe depression and that she may try suicide again."

"You're right. Pain and depression are highly correlated," I say, echoing her concern.

"Complicating things further, she also has a history of cutting and uncontrolled panic attacks that don't seem to respond to the medication we're giving her."

"Sounds like I'll have my work cut out for me."

During our first session, I notice that Julia's physical appearance is rather symbolic. She's of average height and weight, but she's dressed completely in black with a nose piercing and hair cut so short that certain sections stand up like spikes. She's also has it dyed bright red. I learn that her

---

3. Name has been changed.

4. Spinal cord fusion is a surgical procedure to stabilize the spine, alleviate pain, and restore functioning by fusing two or more vertebrae together.

hair color reflects the type of mood she's in. Black is for depression and red is for anxiety and pain.

She also has a number of tattoos that are visible on her neck, chest, wrists, and calves, but there are none on her arms. On those are the scars from her cutting. They run up her skin like military hash marks, and I can see the same markings on her upper legs when she wears shorts.

While I've dealt with other young women who expressed and managed their emotional pain through cutting, I've never seen anything as severe as Julia's case. I can understand why Pam referred her to me. The presence of such intropunitive[5] behavior combined with repeated serious suicide attempts and chronic pain is a devil's brew—not to mention a nightmare to manage on an outpatient basis.

Julia reminds me that this is not her first rodeo, but despite her appearance and bravado, I find her to be quite open.

"Dr. G, I've seen a lot of psychologists over the years. Most of them have been duds, but Dr. Pam says you're different, so I'll give you a try."

Impressed by her frankness, I decide to use her positive relationship with Dr. King to build a therapeutic alliance.

"That seems fair, Julia. Dr. King has told me a lot about you, too, and I think if we work together, I can help," I say, pausing to gauge her reaction. "So, tell me about your pain."

When dealing with a patient who's struggling with chronic pain, I've learned that this is the first topic that must be explored. The human nervous system is so acutely aware of severe pain that it takes priority in a patient's life, influencing nearly every decision they make. If it's not managed effectively, it will prevent the patient from being able to focus on anything else.

---

5. Intropunitive: The tendency to inflict punishment on the oneself.

In comprehensive pain management models, this is accomplished by the physician first prescribing pain medications to reduce the patient's awareness of their pain. Next, they are assigned physical and occupational therapy to improve their mobility. The role of the psychologist in this model is to provide supportive counseling and psychotherapy to address their emotional reactions and to teach psychological coping and pain management strategies.

"When I was pregnant with my son, my back really got worse. I was 20 and after I recovered from giving birth, I began experiencing back spasms and pain in my legs. It got so bad that sometimes my legs would give out on me and I'd fall and not be able to get up. It was scary, especially with an infant son to take care of. I was finally diagnosed with a degenerative disc disease[6]."

"What kind of treatment did you get?"

"Oh, the usual," she responds, sighing. "Physical therapy, muscle relaxants, and shots in my back. I eventually had several back operations, including a fusion. It helped for a while but eventually the pain came back. I learned to live with it. However, when my daughter was born two years ago, it all got worse. I was having trouble walking and even getting out of bed, which was terrible with a newborn as well as another young child. That's when I met Dr. Pam. She's a great doctor and has really helped me. My pain is much better. Now, it only occasionally gets in the way although there are still some days when I have trouble doing anything physical."

"Did any of the other psychologists you saw teach you any

---

6. Degenerative disc disease is a form of arthritis that causes a deterioration in the structure of the spinal joints (discs) resulting in pain and loss of function.

pain management strategies?" I ask, trying to get the bottom of her issues with her psychotherapists.

"No, not really," she says in a flat tone bordering on disgust. "They seemed more interested in other issues like my depression and panic attacks and my cutting myself."

"I see. Well, I'd like to begin by teaching you some psychological pain management strategies if you're interested."

"I would be very interested!" she says with a genuine smile.

Over the next few months, I focus on teaching Julia an array of psychological pain management strategies that complement the medication and the physical and occupational therapy Dr. King has prescribed.

Patients struggling with chronic pain often acknowledge that opiates don't actually remove their pain. They simply reduce one's awareness of it. Similarly, the strategies I'm teaching Julia involve manipulating her awareness of her pain utilizing quasi self-hypnosis.

I first train her in relaxation techniques such as deep and methodical breathing combined with enhanced muscle relaxation along with auditory suggestions, which allow her to enter into a calm and suggestible state. I also help her create a mental cue (i.e., a visual image or a sound) that she can associate with the state of pain-free relaxation to use whenever she needs. Most patients require multiple training sessions to master these skills, but Julia is a quick learner and impresses me not only with her motivation but her ability to process and learn new information quickly.

Between Dr. King's pain management treatment and this training, Julia learns to manage her physical pain successfully within six months. However, despite this huge victory, her depression still lingers.

~

When I walk into the waiting area for our session, Julia is slumped over in a chair in with her hoodie pulled over her head. I'm a bit taken aback since she never wears hoodies. Typically, she prefers jackets or a woolen sweater. She never wears anything to cover her spiked hair.

"Hello, Julia," I say in the same tone I've used for the last six months.

Instead of responding with her usual "Hi, Dr. G!" she simply stands without a word. As we walk into the treatment room, she finds her chair and sits slumped over with the hoodie covering her head. She does not make eye contact.

My first thought is that she may be having a significant increase in her chronic pain.

"Julia, how are you feeling? Is your pain worse?"

"No. It's manageable," she replies tersely before falling silent.

Sometimes when treating a patient, especially when they're clearly upset or struggling, it's important to wait for them to be ready to talk. So, we sit in silence; however, I can feel the tension building between us. Watching her, hood pulled over her head staring at the floor, I can sense that she's desperate to talk but can't find the words. I will have to be the one to break the silence.

"Julia, tell me what's going on. You seem very different today. Has something happened?"

As if a spell were broken, she lifts her head. I can see her face, and there are dark circles under her eyes. While she's not crying, there are remnants of splotchy red spots around her cheeks. Without a word, Julia pushes back the sleeve of her hoodie from her left arm revealing a heavily bandaged wrist.

"I tried to kill myself yesterday," she says.

Words no psychotherapist ever wants to hear.

It's unfortunately not uncommon in outpatient therapy for

depressed patients to experience suicidal ideation. While each occurrence needs to be monitored and taken seriously, such ideation, in my experience, is usually passive, meaning that for some patients, there isn't an active intent or plan to kill themselves. The ideation is an expression of their emotional distress. That's why it's so important to maintain the treatment alliance so that patients feel free to express their thoughts no matter how dark they may be. However, it's a nightmare when a patient has active suicidal ideation or, worse yet, acts on their impulse.

I've had very few patients attempt suicide over the course of my career. When it has occurred, the patient was either early in the treatment process when the therapeutic alliance had not yet been established, or they were undergoing a traumatic life event. More frequently, though, I've found that suicide attempts are often a plea for help rather than an actual death wish[7].

Unfortunately, I've found that when a patient truly wants to kill themselves, there is no way to stop them. They often do not give any warning, and despite there being volumes of books written about the risk factors for suicide, it's generally acknowledged that even experienced clinicians are unable to predict if or when it will occur.

I've only treated two patients who actually succeeded. Both were males. One was a young man in his thirties with paraplegia[8] secondary to a spinal cord injury he sustained in a motor vehicle accident. He suffered from intractable nerve pain that worsened over time. He overdosed on pain medications

---

7. In this context a desire for self-destruction, often accompanied by feelings of depression, hopelessness,
    and self-reproach.
8. Paraplegia: paralysis of the legs and lower body, typically caused by spinal injury or disease.

and wrote in his suicide note that he could no longer tolerate the pain.

The second was a police officer who was caught up in a scandal. He shot himself with his service pistol and wrote in his note that he couldn't face the public disgrace. In both instances, family and peers were shocked since there was no warning. For me, each left a scar as I struggled not just with the sadness of the loss but also the haunting fear that I missed something in their treatment—thoughts that always began *If only I had known, I could have...*

Staring at Julia's bandaged wrist, I can feel my heart beginning to race. I'm concerned because she's clearly suffering, but I also feel apprehensive because, while I know she has a history of suicidal gestures, she hasn't been particularly depressed recently. Clearly something had changed.

While there's no playbook for dealing with this type of event in treatment, a person who attempts suicide generally feels alone in their suffering. The first step to help them is to join them emotionally and empathize with the distress that's driving the behavior.

"Julia, you must have been feeling terrible to try that. How are you feeling now?"

"Kind of numb and sort of foolish if I am being honest because it didn't change anything. Every time I've done this, it's always the same. I get myself all worked up, do something like this, and, in the end, I just feel empty."

"Is that what you're feeling now? Empty?"

She looks up and makes eye contact with me for the first time in the session, but I see a flash of another emotion cross her face.

"And angry!" she shouts.

"Angry?" I ask.

"Yeah, at myself, Dr. G. What's wrong with me? When am I ever going to learn?"

"Well, perhaps we can figure this out together," I say, remaining calm.

Julia sits up in her chair and pushes back the hood from her face.

"My dad came back for one of his unannounced visits last weekend."

"Tell me what happened, Julia," I say, sensing she's ready to talk.

"It's always the same with him ever since he left us when I was a kid. He just shows up at the house once or twice a year acting like he never left. I'm never sure when he will show up, but when he does, he's full of energy and religious talk. Sometimes when he was high on cocaine, things were really crazy. It was like a storm, and everything became chaotic. Before she joined AA, my mother would get upset when he came home and would drink more. They would fight, but she always let him stay. I didn't care if it was crazy, though. I waited for those visits. I just wanted us to be a family again like before he left."

"How long does he typically stay?"

"Only a day or two. In the past, it depended a lot on whether he and Mom got into a fight, but even if they didn't, he would always leave abruptly without saying goodbye. That was the worst for me. I'd get so depressed. The feeling of loss is unbearable, and I feel so empty that I just want to die. Sometimes when I was younger, I'd cut myself after he left just to feel some relief. When I was older, I drank and used drugs if I could get them. Sometimes I'd overdose and end up in the hospital."

"Is that what happened this time?"

Julia doesn't respond to my question immediately. Her

eyes, however, begin to well up with tears. She wipes them away with the sleeve of her hoodie.

"No. This time was worse than the others. Normally, he just disappears without saying anything, like a ghost, but this time for some reason, as he was getting ready to leave, he got himself all worked up. Started praying out loud and then he yelled at me, telling me that I was a bad person, a sinner and that no one like me could be his daughter. He then said that he was leaving because he couldn't be around someone like me who was going to go to hell. Then, he stormed off into the night. I was devastated. He was telling me that he was leaving because of me."

"Those are terrible things to say to someone, especially to your child. Is this when you began to feel suicidal?"

"No, it's what I did after he left that triggered me."

"What did you do next?"

Julia lowers her head, shaking it slowly.

"Oh God, Dr. G! I am such a fool. After he left, I was so upset, crying and having all these mixed-up feelings—sad, angry, guilty. I kept thinking that he was right, and I was bad. That his leaving us and his comings and goings were all somehow my fault. I felt so alone. I just wanted to be with someone. I just wanted to be held. I needed to be held. So, I called one of the guys I've been seeing and asked if I could come over and be with him."

"So, you went to see him?"

"Yes."

"And then what happened?"

"We had sex. But afterward, when I wanted to stay, he told me I had to leave. That's when the bottom dropped out for me. Sitting in my car in front of his apartment, I felt so used and so empty and alone. I suddenly couldn't breathe, and my head was spinning. I just wanted all the thoughts and feelings running through my head to stop, so I took a razor blade from the glove compartment and slashed my wrist. Then, there was blood everywhere and I got scared and realized that I didn't want to die. I drove myself to the ER. Told them some cock-and-bull story about cutting myself on a broken window. I'm not sure they believed me, but it was really late, so they just stitched me up and let me go."

When a patient discusses suicide ideation or a past suicide attempt, they generally experience a sense of relief the moment they share these thoughts with their therapist. However, the effects of this catharsis[9] tend to be short-lived. The real work around the issue of suicidal ideation or the act itself is to build a stable therapeutic infrastructure for the patient to be able to manage these thoughts and impulses.

One frequently asked question I receive is when or *if* to hospitalize the patient. From my experience, if the patient has recently tried to commit suicide and continues with suicidal ideation, hospitalization is usually needed so that they can be in a controlled and supportive environment that allows time for the impulse to subside. In these cases, voluntary admission is always preferable since involuntary hospitalization can disrupt the therapeutic alliance with the patient. Unfortunately, though, if a patient is determined to kill themselves, while hospitalization may delay the inevitable, it does not prevent the event from occurring once the patient is discharged.

In Julia's case, I don't feel that hospitalization is the most effective option, primarily because her suicidal impulse has passed and she's no longer preoccupied with killing herself. Like many patients, she feels ashamed and depressed after the

---

9. Catharsis: the process of releasing, and thereby providing relief from, strong or repressed emotions.

attempt, not determined to kill herself. She's still psychologically fragile, though, so I decide to increase the level of support in her treatment.

"Julia, you've been through an emotional meat grinder in the last few days. We've been concentrating on managing your pain up until now, but I think it's time to focus on what's been driving your depression. Do you agree?"

Breaking eye contact, she stares at her hands for several moments. I feel uncertain as to what this silence means since she doesn't respond to my suggestion, so I wait, hoping that I've not just become another "dud" in her long line of psychologists.

"I guess that would be okay," she says, lifting her head. "Yeah, Dr. G, I'd like to do that. I don't want to feel like this anymore."

"Good. The first thing I would like to do with you is to temporally increase the frequency of treatment. You've been coming in weekly for a while, but how about if you come in three times a week for the next two weeks to focus intensely on this recent occurrence. Then, if you are feeling better, we can resume weekly sessions."

"I think I'd like that."

"I'd also like to get Dr. King involved. Again, she's been primarily focused on managing your pain, but I think some changes in your medications can help with your depression."

Julia hesitates for a moment. "Do you think she'll be upset with me over my cutting myself?"

"Julia, she's your doctor, and it's nothing she hasn't seen or dealt with before. I think she'll be more concerned about your well-being. Also, I'll explain it to her. Think of us as all being a part of your treatment team. Our goal is for you to feel better and deal with this issue."

She exhales and sits up straight.

"Finally, there's one more thing I'm going to ask you to do. It's important to have your whole support system involved in your treatment. I know that you are very close to your mother and your aunt. I want you to discuss with them what you've been going through. It's very important that you not be alone with your feelings."

Julia smiles for the first time during this session.

"Oh, they know. Who do you think I called to get me from the ER? They were pretty upset with me, but we talked a lot last night. They are the ones who urged me to talk with you. So, no problem. They are definitely on board."

As our session draws to a close, I take out my business card, write my private number on the back, and hand it to her.

"Julia, we are in this together. This is my private number. If you are ever feeling suicidal again, or you just feel that you need to talk things through, call me."

Most of my peers would feel that giving Julia my personal number is controversial. Their argument would be that I'm fostering patient dependency. However, my experience is different. This is not a general strategy that I use with every patient but rather one that's based on my assessment of an individual's clinical needs for support. The patients who've had my number in the past rarely called me, and when they did, it was to diffuse a legitimate crisis that fostered their progress in treatment. I've also found this strategy useful in addressing feelings of emotional isolation. Similar to patients who have panic attacks, reassurance often comes from simply knowing they have their medications with them. Even if they don't take them, knowing they have access can ward off the onset of the attack.

～

Julia's suicide attempt begins the next phase of her treatment. We focus on addressing her depression and work with Dr. King to find the appropriate concoction of psychotropic medications that will address her neurochemical exhaustion[10] caused by her childhood trauma, dysfunctional relationships, and her chronic pain. This process involves a trial-and-error approach. Much like Dr. Ormiston's strategy with the NBI patients, effective pain management, often requires considerable precision in the combinations of mood regulating, neuroinhibitory[11], and anxiolytic medications[12]. It's a constant reminder that pain and depression are complex neurological as well as neuropsychological events.

While Dr. King stabilizes the medication, it becomes my role to address the psychological issues underlying her depression and suicide attempt. This involves helping her connect the impact of her dysfunctional relationship with her father to her behavior.

With Julia's permission, I start exploring the dynamics of her depression by digging deeper into her developmental history.

"Julia, I'd like you to tell me more about yourself. What was it like for you growing up?"

"Dr. G, I come from a very crazy family," she says, staring straight into my eyes. "My mom told me that my dad suffered from bipolar disorder and cocaine addiction and that he'd had multiple psychiatric hospitalizations. During one of his episodes, he had some sort of a 'religious epiphany' and became a street preacher, which was when he left us. I was so young that I don't remember any of it. He eventually ended up

---

10. Neurochemical exhaustion refers to decreases in the concentration of neurotransmitters within the central nervous system.
11. Medication that inhibits activity in the nervous system.
12. Medication that reduces anxiety.

living mostly in Oklahoma, but I remember that he would occasionally return home for short periods of time."

My mind flashes back to Mike and his religious mania.

"He would just show up out of the blue and maybe stay for a day or two, acting like he'd never left. He was always dressed in black and wearing a large silver crucifix around his neck. My mom would let him stay, but these visits upset her, and she would drink more when he was around. You couldn't really have a conversation with him because he was always ranting about God and the Bible. None of it made sense to me, but I was always glad to see him because he was my dad. Then, for no apparent reason, he would just abruptly disappear without saying goodbye. I remember that I would sit by the window in the front room of our house for days after he left waiting for him to come home."

"How did this make you feel, Julia?"

"I remember feeling sad all the time, longing for him to come back, but when he did, he would inevitably leave again. I loved him. Still do. I think I'm still waiting for him to come home and stay even though I know he's not going to."

I find myself having to control the sadness and anger bubbling within me. Both as a clinician and an investigator, I've seen the depths of human perversity, and, unfortunately, I still don't have an answer for the behavior Julia's father exhibits. I hold the relationships I have with my wife and children sacred. The thought of abandoning them—for any reason—is so incomprehensible and disturbing to me that I'm unable to treat such individuals that do this although I regularly treat the problems their actions create in others.

"Because my dad was gone, I was raised primarily by my mom and my aunt," Julia continues.

Julia shares that both her mother and aunt suffered from alcoholism and that their ability to parent Julia was erratic.

Left virtually unsupervised in her early adolescence, she began using drugs and alcohol and became sexually promiscuous. She also started cutting herself. Julia eventually stopped using drugs and alcohol in her mid-twenties when, with the help of her mother and aunt, she found her way into the AA program.

"My entire family is in AA except my father. My mother and all of my aunts and uncles are in the program. We sometimes attend meetings together. AA saved my life," she says.

As Julia describes her family dynamics, I become convinced that while her chronic pain is an exacerbating factor in her depression, it's the dysfunctional nature of her codependency with her father that's the core issue of her behavior.

"Julia, how do you feel when your father shows up now?" I ask.

A brief expression of pain crosses her face.

"At first, I feel elated. In fact, I will drop everything I'm doing, even send the kids to my mom's or my aunt's, just to spend time with him. But his visits are the same just like when I was a child. He stays for a while and then departs, and when he leaves, it feels like the bottom of my world is dropping out. I feel this empty feeling in my gut and need to find some way to fill it or at least stop it."

"What would you do to stop it?"

Pausing, Julia moves around restlessly in her chair.

"You know, Dr. G, I used to cut myself. It took the feelings away for a while, but I don't do that anymore. Also, when I was in high school, I would use sex to get attention from the boys. It made me feel wanted for a moment, but when they would drop me, I'd feel really bad."

Curious about her current relationships, I ask, "What about the guys you're seeing now?"

"Oh, I don't do one-night stands anymore, but I guess the

pattern is the same with them although it somehow it feels different."

"Different? What do you mean?"

"It starts out fine and I feel that I love them and that they love me, but then they just leave. It's like there's something wrong with me—that I'm not good enough for them to stay."

Suddenly, her facial expression changes, and I can see she is making a mental connection between her behavior and her father.

"It makes me feel just like when Dad would leave."

"Yes, there is a connection to your relationship with your father," I say, reinforcing her insight. "Like you are trying to fill in the emotional void he creates when he leaves."

Psychotherapy has been described as a process of peeling back layers in which deeper emotional truths are gradually revealed. However, it's not a process void of emotional distress. Thankfully, though, one of the benefits of long-term therapy is that the patient has a safe and supportive environment to explore these issues, which lessens the inner conflict. Over time, treatment allows them to integrate their insights into their sense of self and ultimately change the way they behave.

Julia shows up to our next treatment session feeling elated.

"Well, Dr. G, Dad visited again and followed the pattern we've been talking about. Just showed up unannounced and then abruptly left again."

"Yes, Julia, that is the pattern we've been discussing."

Then, smiling like the *Cheshire cat* from Lewis Carroll's *Alice's Adventures in Wonderland* she says, "Dr. G, when he left this time without even saying goodbye, I remembered our discussion about how I'm always waiting for him to come back and realized that it's been the same cycle my whole life. How I would fall asleep crying by the window late at night waiting for him. How I felt that he left because there was something wrong with me. That I somehow wasn't good enough for him to stay, and if I could get him to, it would fix things. Fix me. Fix him."

We've had similar conversations before, but Julia's expression this time is different.

"When I met with him this time, all those discussions we've had in therapy about my relationship with him ran through my mind. It was like I understood who he really was for the first time. That all his comings and goings were about some need in him and not about some failing in me. I realized that he will always be this way. He is driven by all his own crazy demons, not by something about me, and I have to start accepting that."

Suddenly, she stops speaking and I remain silent. I have to give her time to process her own insight.

"As I thought about what we've been talking about and the idea of acceptance," she continues, "that anxious feeling I always felt when he showed up was gone. I suddenly knew I was done waiting and done fixing. A saying we have in AA is that when we have an unsolvable problem, we have to give it to God. This came to me, and I knew that's what I have to do with Dad."

I nod in agreement, allowing her space to process and think.

"And, oh, by the way, you know those assholes I've been dating? Well, I'm going to stop letting them use me. I thought I wasn't good enough for them or that I didn't measure up, but I can see what you've been saying about the similarities in my relationship with them and my father—how I've been trying to fix what I felt about myself and him through them."

This session is a significant turning point in Julia's treatment. Our explorations of the connection between her sense of self, her father's erratic visits, and her relationship with men are now clear to her. We now can start brainstorming ideas about how to best handle her father's unexpected visits and her relationship with her boyfriends.

Much of this involves setting boundaries. With her father, since she still wants to maintain their relationship, she has to limit the amount of time she spends with him and stay committed to her routine even if he visits unexpectedly. In her romantic relationships, she has to slow down the speed of intimacy so that she doesn't become physically and emotionally attached until she knows the other person's intentions. Easier said than done, of course.

There are ups and downs during this phase as she struggles to develop these behaviors into habits. This is especially true with her boyfriends.

"Dr. G, it's so frustrating," she says slamming her fists against the arm rests. "I can do what we've talked about with my dad pretty well, but with the guys, my emotions get all muddled. It's like I hear us talking about what to do in my head, but I can't seem to slow things down."

Learning to take back one's sense of self-worth is never an easy process.

"Julia, it's the early days yet. You're managing your father better, and that's progress. With the guys, it's probably going to take more work. It's triggering lots of different emotions, not just ones related to your father. These will be more difficult to sort out. Again, just keep trying to slow things down, and remember, that with them, it's about controlling your feelings so you can get enough information about theirs."

As Julia leaves my office, I notice that she has a slightly

hunched posture, indicating that she lacks confidence. This is difficult for me to see.

"Julia, sometimes therapy is two steps forward and one step back," I say before she leaves. "But I know that with practice, you'll get better."

During our next session she's much more positive.

"I was out with this guy the other night," she says, smiling. This time, however, her smile isn't giddy. It carries a breath of confidence. "It was our first date," she continues, "and he wanted to get intimate. I said that I wasn't ready, and he pretty much lost interest in me at that point, and our date ended, but I felt good about it. He'd failed the asshole test. The funny thing is that I heard your voice in my head telling me to go slow the whole time."

The underlying goal of therapy is for the patient to internalize the insights they've learned into their sense of self. In my experience, there are several stages to this process. First, the patient identifies the underlying causes of their problem. Next, they devise strategies to address them. Then, finally, they attempt to integrate what they've learned into their daily life through a process of trial and error. Patients often experience frustration at not being able to utilize the strategies effectively in the beginning as they feel awkward or clumsy. This is when the psychotherapist steps into help the patient to cope with their frustration and to encourage their efforts.

If the patient perseveres, they almost always experience a breakthrough. This is when the therapist must reinforce their success so that the patient's actions become fully integrated into their sense of self. Like a child learning to walk, they have not yet owned their newfound abilities and still require external support. Many patients remain at this stage.

Ideally, though, the patient will fully integrate the strategies into their lives by the end of treatment. Like a professional musician or athlete who after extensive practice executes a behavior with automaticity, the patient will now be able to make decisions that align with what matters to them the most, almost without thinking.

~

When Julia and I meet again, I'm stunned as to how far she's come. She sits down in the same chair that she was slumped over in months ago with a new sense of poise and confidence.

"Dr. G, things are going well," she says. "My dad still comes and goes as always, but it doesn't upset me the way it used to. Sometimes I see him, sometimes not, depending on what else I have to do. I don't feel like I'm waiting for him anymore. Actually, I just feel bad for him. He's just so crazy, but that's not my circus. Also, I have a new boyfriend, Gary. We've been out on a few dates, but I am taking it slow with him, like we've discussed, and he was okay with that. It's letting us both get to know each other."

"It seems like you've figured some things out. How does that make you feel?"

"Makes me feel confident. Like I finally know how to manage both them and my feelings. Don't feel like I'm riding that emotional roller coaster anymore. I'm grateful for your help, Dr. G. You're a great listener and have always been there for me."

The fluidity with which she implements the strategies she's learned suggests that she's integrated them into her core identity. She rarely mentions them as a part of a conscious effort anymore. They are a permanent part of her coping repertoire.

~

With Julia's chronic pain and depressive episodes under control, I turn my attention to her panic attacks, which continue to perplex me. Based on her description, they occur at regular intervals, but I haven't been able to identify any specific triggers connected with them. Adding to my frustration, none of the medications that Dr. King has prescribed, including powerful anxiolytics, can control them and my meditation and relaxation strategies are also ineffective.

Julia and I discuss this during our next session. The conversation flows as normal with her sharing the ups and downs of her life, but I still can't discern a potential trigger. As I listen deeply to the sound of her voice, hoping to pick up on a slight tone shift, anything that will help me, she suddenly stops speaking and stares into space. Other than breathing deeply, Julia's completely detached from everything around her.

"Julia?" I ask.

"Julia?"

She continues to stare blankly without speaking. This lasts for about 90 seconds. She then shakes her head and refocuses on the session but is mildly confused and disoriented.

"Julia, what just happened?" I ask, thinking she had a traumatic flashback.

"Oh, I just had a panic attack," she responds casually while adjusting her seating position.

"Really? Are they always like that?"

"Well, yes. Sort of, sometimes longer, I think."

Suddenly, I realize that Julia had reported having frequent panic attacks, but I never received a detailed description of them or actually witnessed her having one. What I just observed is not like a typical panic attack. It is, however, similar to partial complex seizures, particularly ones involving a brief loss of consciousness that I've observed with brain-injured patients.

"Julia, I've seen a lot of panic attacks during my career, but what you just had looked much more like a seizure. Have you ever had seizures?"

"Yeah, when I was a kid," she responds nonchalantly.

Julia shares that when she was five years old, she fell down a flight of stairs in her home and fractured her skull. A few months later, her mother noticed that she was having episodes where she would briefly stare off into space. Her mother took her to her pediatrician who referred her to a pediatric neurologist. There, she was diagnosed with partial complex seizures and placed on medication.

As Julia relates the history of her seizures, her body posture stiffens, and she wraps her arms around her stomach.

"I was on seizure medications until I was 13. They seemed to be able to control my episodes, but when I was 13, I started seeing a new doctor. Since I hadn't had any seizures for a while, he told me I didn't need the medication anymore and took me off them. For a while I was okay, but when I turned 14, I began having episodes again."

"What happened then?"

"The new doctor referred me to a psychiatrist. That's when I was diagnosed as having panic attacks. He put me on Xanax."

"Did the Xanax ever stop the panic attacks?"

Julia's eyes well up with tears, and she begins to sob.

"No, the panic attacks never got under control. Since I received the diagnosis, I have been in and out of treatment with half a dozen psychiatrists, all of whom eventually gave up trying to control them. Some even accused me of abusing their medications or of being noncompliant, which I wasn't."

I pause to give her chance to process her emotions and hand her a tissue.

"Julia, I think it's quite possible that you haven't been having panic attacks at all. I think you still may be having those seizures you had as a child. Let me see what I can do to straighten this out."

Her arms relax as she nods her head.

After the session, I consult with Dr. King. She helps me set up a referral with the Medical College of Wisconsin Neurology Department for a seizure evaluation, and a month later, the results come back positive for partial complex seizures. In consultation with one of their neurologists, she places her on a seizure medication called Keppra, and Julia's "panic attacks" completely stop after a few dosage adjustments to her medication.

When Julia arrives to my office, she states that her seizures have stopped, and I can see the look of relief on her face.

"Julia, how are you feeling now that you know that what they called panic attacks are actually partial complex seizures?"

"Dr. G, it feels like a great weight has been taken off me," she replies, smiling brightly.

"This is significant, Julia," I say, feeling her sense of relief.

Sitting back in her chair, she runs her hands through her hair, which today is in its natural brown color.

"I know, Dr. G. I am so relieved that we know the cause of what's been happening to me, and that it's something from a physical injury that can be treated! For so long, I thought these episodes meant that I was emotionally broken and unfixable—like there was something deeply wrong with me as a person. It made me doubt myself and the progress I've made. It's like I'm just discovering the real me."

This misdiagnosis of Julia's partial complex seizures as panic attacks reminds me of an observation Harry Stacks Sullivan made in his book *The Psychiatric Interview*, which I read when I was a government investigator dreaming of going to graduate school for psychotherapy. He acknowledged that psychiatric and physical symptoms can interact and that physical symptoms can be expressions of psychological distress. He also cautioned that neither patient nor doctor should ever conclude that a symptom is purely psychological until all the possible physical causes have been ruled out. This is why Sullivan always insisted that his patients complete a physical before their first appointment.

～

Hanging on the wall of my consulting office is an 18-inch by 24-inch framed and mounted 1000-piece jigsaw puzzle. The image is a copy of a famous Norman Rockwell painting entitled *Doctor and the Doll* in which a white-haired doctor places a stethoscope on a doll being held up by a young girl dressed in a red beret, coat, scarf, and plaid skirt. It was given to me by Julia during our last session after four years of therapy.

The moment she handed me the painting was an emotional one for the both of us since it signified both the journey and the end of our work together. Such moments are bittersweet for me. In working with patients long term, I feel a fondness for them as fellow travelers on our shared human journey. With Julia, there's a lingering sadness that the journey has come to an end, but I feel a sense of gratitude and excitement about her evolution into a capable and confident young woman.

Holding out the gift in the palm of her hands, Julia smiles and her eyes water.

"Dr. G, I wanted to give you this to thank you for everything you've done for me. You hung in there with me and helped me figure things out. I feel so different than when I first came to see you. I'm not in pain like I was, and I'm not riding a roller coaster of constant ups and downs. I feel more in control of my life."

Unwrapping the gift, I see it's a jigsaw puzzle of the Rockwell image, and I'm suddenly brought to tears. Julia's thoughtfulness is not lost on me, and, in such moments, I find that my emotions are difficult to put into words.

"Thank you, Julia. This is a lovely gift," I say, holding it up. "It must have taken a lot of effort to put it together and get it framed. The Rockwell image is beautiful."

"You're welcome, Dr. G."

"Julia, you've worked very hard in therapy, and I can clearly see the changes in you."

Julia smiles broadly and sits a little straighter in her chair.

Any present a therapist receives at the end of treatment is called a termination gift. The giver's intent is to share their gratitude, but I also believe that the gifts themselves carry symbolic value.

Julia's choice of a 1000-piece puzzle is symbolic to me because she would do puzzles as a coping strategy when she was upset or stressed. She told me that the distraction they provided calmed her down, which I found fascinating because, if I were to do them, I would actually become more anxious, not less. But this was one of her coping mechanisms that she used prior to treatment with me. As I got to know Julia, I began to feel that these puzzles represented more than just a distraction from her problems. More accurately, they captured her innate resilience. She was, after all, a survivor who always found a way to put herself back together piece by piece.

To me, the puzzle also symbolized the treatment process. With Julia, her challenges were like the intricate pieces of a puzzle that we had to put together until a clear image emerged. The first part of the puzzle involved understanding the intricate layers of her relationship with her father. The second was her desire for stability in the form of a masculine figure in her romantic relationships with the final piece being the misdiagnosis of her seizures as panic attacks.

As I look at the painting in my hands, I'm intrigued by the possible transferential[13] father-daughter element between us in the Rockwell painting.

"Julia, why did you choose this Rockwell painting?" I ask, curious.

"Oh, Dr. G, because that's us. You are the doctor. I am the girl, and the doll is the broken part of me that you fixed."

I'm tempted to say—That *you* fixed. While I may have been the one helping her navigate her situations, she was the one who put in the hard work to make the necessary changes. Wiping the tears from my eyes, I decide not to, recognizing that she already owns her progress. We sit in silence contemplating the puzzle, our journey together, and all of the emotions that have transpired between us. As my thoughts drift, I can't help but think that the dysfunction of her father's coming and going caused her so much pain. His own mental health issues led her down a dark and desperate path, causing her to doubt herself and nearly end her life. This is especially hard for me to contemplate as a father. My own son, who's now fully recovered from his illness thanks to numerous stays at the Mayo Clinic and consultations with specialists, never spent a single day wondering where I was or whether I'd return to him. Julia, on the other hand, spent her entire childhood (and even some of her adulthood) longing for her father hoping that he would stay for good. My son never sat by the window with tears in his eyes waiting for me to come home. In

---

13. Relating to transference, the act of re-experiencing within psychotherapy with the therapist feelings or desires originally experienced in childhood with respect to a parent.

contrast, Julia searched for fatherly devotion and protective affection in every uncaring man she met. Having been by my son every step of his journey, I cannot fathom how a parent leaves their child to pass through the gauntlet alone.

Questions for Consideration

1. How do you think the author's situation with his son impacted him professionally and emotionally in his treatment with Julia? How do you think the stress of dealing with his son's serious illness affected, complicated, and/or enhanced his treatment methods?

2. Do you think the author's treatment mirrored a parental figure and how they would guide their own child through some of these complex relationships? Why do you think Julia heard the author's voice when dealing with her situations with men rather than her mother's or aunt's or her own?

3. Should her mother and aunt have played a more significant role when her father left without explaining what was happening? How did her mother's alcoholism impact Julia in her adolescent years? Was that a contributing factor to some of the other mental health issues that she had?

4. Why didn't her mother ask additional questions when the doctor took her off her seizure medication? Could it have been financial?

5. Why did the author tell Julia to reach out to her mother after her suicide attempt? Why was that important?

6. If Julia didn't trust her family members to support her, how might the situation have turned out differently?

7. Why do you think that Julia never used the author's personal number? Was it solely an emotional safety net? Did having it feel similar to a security blanket?

8. Do you think Julia finally learned how to protect herself and her peace? Do you believe that she developed true respect for herself? How do you think seeing her in this condition impacted her two children?

THE DESPERATE DEPORTEE

"Give me your tired, your poor, your huddled masses yearning to breathe free."

— EMMA LAZARUS

Widener University
Chester, Pennsylvania, 2004

As I sit nervously in the waiting area of Dean Virginia Braebender's office at Widener University's Institute for Graduate Clinical Psychology, I'm fighting off the effects of jet lag. Having just gotten off the red-eye from San Francisco to Philadelphia, I can feel exhaustion tugging at the edges of my capacity for attention. My mental fog, however, is quickly interrupted by the secretary.

"The dean will see you now," she says, ushering me into a book-lined office.

I enter the office slowly, noticing that the spring sunlight is streaming through a large window facing the university's grass-covered quad. A woman with shoulder-length brown hair and bangs stands up in a formal manner and offers her hand to me.

"Good morning, Dr. Gillespie. I'm Virginia Braebender."

"It's nice to finally meet you in person, Dean Braebender," I reply, shaking her hand.

She invites me to sit before returning to her chair behind a large wooden desk covered with neatly piled stacks of papers. Looking at her desk, she starts perusing the vitae[1] that I sent over a few days ago. An old anxious feeling presses into my consciousness. I feel like I'm back in school watching my teacher evaluate my term paper. That is, until she looks up at me and smiles warmly.

"Dr. Exner thinks quite highly of you, and I think quite highly of his judgment. We have worked on a number of projects together for the Society for Personality Assessment over the years, especially on the Rorschach test."

My anxiety dissipates as the introductory pleasantries gradually fade into the background.

"He mentored me during my graduate training at Long Island University," I confirm. "Taught me how to do scientific research. We published a study of the stability of Rorschach subject's responses over time. He also helped me get my internship at Newington and recommended me for my postdoc residency in Massachusetts, and we've stayed in contact over the years."

---

1. Vitae refers to a *curriculum vitae*, a brief biographical résumé of one's professional career and training.

She interlaces her fingers together and places her elbows on her desk. Apparently, the pleasantries are now officially over.

"He also tells me that you have experience doing startups and thinks you'd be a good fit for what I want to do here."

"Yes, when I met with him at the conference in Los Angeles, he told me you were thinking of creating a neuropsychology clinic here at the university and are looking for a neuropsychologist with experience in building clinical programs," I say, maintaining a formal tone.

She allows me to continue. I briefly discuss my work with Dr. Ormiston at Bethesda and the NBI. I also describe the process of building a private practice in Wisconsin with Dr. King and more recently in Silicon Valley. However, what I don't mention is that this meeting, which has been set in motion by our colleague John E. Exner Junior, who's a distinguished scientist[2] and a master of the Rorschach inkblot test[3], was the result of a chance encounter at a hotel bar in Los Angeles. He was presenting at a conference I attended, and, over two

---

2. For a respected academic research scientist who received the 1997 American Psychological Association's Award for Distinguished Professional Contributions to Applied Research in 1997, Dr. Exner's career had an unusual course. Rather than attending college directly after high school, he enlisted in the Army as a private and served during World War II. Rising to the rank of sergeant, he became one of the "Flying Sergeants," noncommissioned enlisted personnel who flew transport aircraft during World War II and again in Korea where he was injured in a crash. It was while recovering at an Army hospital that he was administered the Rorschach test and became fascinated with it. After being discharged, he completed his undergraduate degree on the GI bill and finished his doctoral dissertation on the test at Cornell University, which became the subsequent focus of his professional career.

3. The Rorschach inkblot test is a psychological test developed by Hermann Rorschach, a Swiss psychiatrist in 1921, in which the subject is presented with 10 ambiguous inkblots and their responses are analyzed to measure their personality characteristics and emotional functioning using psychological interpretation and complex scientifically derived algorithms.

scotches, I confided in him that I was in a professional transition and looking for work in the Philadelphia area. He placed an early morning phone call to Dr. Braebender that set this meeting into motion.

"Why are you moving from California to Pennsylvania?" she asks, seeming satisfied with this summary of my professional background.

"My wife Astrid is a human resources and labor lawyer and has just been promoted to the senior vice president at the *Philadelphia Inquirer*," I reply.

She nods, indicating that I should offer more clarification.

"As I mentioned, I left Bethesda and opened my practice in Wisconsin when my eldest son became seriously ill. After he recovered, Astrid was offered a position that was too good to pass up with the Knight Ridder newspaper company's flagship paper the *San Jose Mercury News* in California. So, we moved the family there, and I began commuting long distance, halfway across the country, in fact, between my Wisconsin practice and a new practice with a psychiatrist partner at El Camino Hospital in Silicon Valley. That commute, while stressful, was doable. However, a transcontinental commute between California and Philadelphia isn't, and that's why I'm here looking for a position in Philadelphia."

Satisfied with my explanation, Dr. Braebender releases her intertwined fingers, and presses both of her forearms against the rests on her chair.

"Let me tell you what I am proposing to do. My department has just received a large federal grant, and I want to use the funds to create a clinic here to train our neuropsychology graduate students to provide low-cost assessments to the local community here in Chester. It's one of the poorest in the state of Pennsylvania."

She pauses for a moment and purses her lips. Her pensive

expression indicates that she is carefully choosing her next words. After a few moments, she finally makes eye contact again.

"I have two very bright neuropsychologists in my department: Dr. Ken Goldberg, who is a tenured professor and is in charge of our neuropsychology training track, and Dr. Mary Lazar whom I've hired to direct the new clinic. She graduated from the neuropsychology track here and has just completed her residency with a specialization in children, which is a service the community really needs. Between them, I believe they can eventually manage and run the facility and the student staff when it's finally up and running, but they don't have any program development experience, let alone building a clinical operation from scratch, and I'm looking for someone who does to help them build it."

I nod and remain silent before she leans forward and places both her elbows on her desk.

"Dr. Gillespie, I want you to be in charge of building it. We have already identified a building on campus that you can have a free hand in redesigning from the ground up. I want you to design everything from the physical layout of the clinic to its fiscal and day-to-day clinical operations. Ken can help you navigate the political pitfalls in dealing with the university's bureaucracy, and, ultimately, once it's up and running, Mary and you will split the clinical work of supervising the students with her handling the children and you the adults. You would be the associate director and an assistant clinical professor in our department here at the university."

What an unexpectedly intriguing idea! Images of Charlie Ormiston, Bethesda, and the NBI flash through my head, and I can feel my heart rate increasing not with anxiety but growing excitement.

Breaking into my reverie, Dr. Braebender says, "I've

arranged for you to have lunch with Ken and Mary, and for us to meet back here later this afternoon, so you can tell me what you think before you fly back to California."

"Sounds good to me," I say, preparing to leave.

"Oh! By the way, we're going to name it the Neuropsychology Assessment Center or *NAC* for short."

NBI...NAC...Program Development...Weird coincidence...Or is it fate?

Later that afternoon, I return to Dr. Braebender's office after my lunch with Ken and Mary.

"So how did it go?" she asks excitedly.

"Fantastic. I like them. It was both a very pleasant and productive lunch. You're right. They are bright neuropsychologists. We not only have a common vision for the new clinic but also have similar views about how to use neuropsychology in treatment. I definitely believe we can work together on this project."

"That's exactly what they said when they called me after meeting with you. Somehow, based on our brief conversations over the phone these past few weeks, I thought you would hit it off. So, what do you think of my proposal? Are you interested?"

"Oh yes! I'm in. Let's build a clinic," I say, closing the deal with a handshake.

Neuropsychology Assessment Center
Chester, Pennsylvania, 2006

It's the beginning of my third year as the Associate Director of NAC, and the center is fully operational and running smoothly. Making it both a viable and valuable resource for students while providing low-cost assessments and treatment for patients has been both professionally and personally reward-ing. However, with the startup development complete, I now mostly just supervise the graduate students, which is causing a feeling of intense malaise at not working with patients directly.

As I enter my office on the second floor this blasé Monday morning, there's a light blinking on my answering machine.

This is likely a message from Ken or Mary wanting to talk about an assessment or administrative issue.

But after pushing the button, I'm surprised to hear an unfamiliar voice.

"Dr. Gillespie, my name is Jacqueline Wright[4]. I'm a legal aid attorney in Valley Forge, Pennsylvania, and I need your assistance. I'm representing an indigent man whose life is in danger due to a miscarriage of justice. Please call me as soon as possible. This is an urgent matter."

Quite the pitch.

Jolted from my stupor, I rush to pick up the receiver and return her call.

"Hello this is Jacqueline Wright," a bright, friendly voice answers.

"Good morning, Ms. Wright. This is Dr. Gillespie from the Widener Neuropsychology Assessment Center. You called earlier with an urgent matter about a client. How can I be of assistance?"

"Oh! I'm so glad you returned my call! I'm desperate and your clinic is my last resort," she says, becoming noticeably more animated.

She explains that her client is a 24-year-old Haitian man

---

4. Name has been changed.

named Claude[5] who's incarcerated in a U.S. Immigration and Customs Enforcement's (ICE) detention facility in Valley Forge awaiting deportation to Haiti.

"Dr. Gillespie, as you are probably aware, legal aid represents indigent clients who could not otherwise afford an attorney. I was contacted for help by Claude's aunt who told me that he had just been discharged from state prison for having robbed a liquor store, and, since he's undocumented, is about to be deported to Haiti where he was born. She's worried that he will not survive his deportation because he was brought here as a baby and has never really lived in Haiti and has no family there. He also does not speak the language, and as his aunt put it, 'He's a sweet boy, but he's not too smart.'"

"So, your client is an undocumented felon who is about to be deported?" I reply, skeptical and puzzled.

"Well, that's not exactly accurate. He is more like a dreamer[6]. His parents brought him to the United States from Haiti when he was one, but both died in a car accident when he was three. His aunt, who was his only living relative in the States, took him in, but neither she nor he ever applied for him to become a citizen. As to his being a felon, I'm not sure that's accurate either."

"Because?" I ask, still confused.

"Because after talking with him and reviewing the court records, what I found is a legal travesty!"

"A legal travesty?" I repeat.

"Yes! Because of what is and is *not* in the court records."

"Which is what exactly?"

"Well, what's in the record is pretty terse and straight

---

5. Name has been changed.

6. A *dreamer* is an individual who is not a US citizen and who has lived in the US without official authorization since coming to the country as a minor.

forward," she says, measuring her words carefully. "Claude was working as a day laborer with the two other defendants. The state alleged that after work on a Friday, they stuck up a liquor store. While it was the other two defendants who went into the store, threatened, and robbed the manager, Claude waited outside. They told the police and assistant district attorney who prosecuted the case that it was Claude who thought up and planned the whole thing. With his two accomplices pointing the finger at Claude and willing to be the state's witnesses, the public defender made a deal with the prosecutor. Claude got three years in state prison, and the others were placed on probation and walked."

I've seen plenty of sloppy legal work in my years as an investigator, but based on her summary, I still don't understand why she feels this is a legal travesty.

"He plead out. What makes this a legal travesty and a miscarriage of justice?" I ask.

Her voice takes on an edge of indignation.

"Because, while I'm not a trained psychologist, when I interviewed him, it was clear to me, and I think would have been clear to anyone including the prosecutor and Claude's public defender, that he was not only 'not too smart' but severely impaired intellectually. So impaired that he not only lacked the mental capacity to understand the plea bargain that he was offered but the crime he was charged with and its consequences. He couldn't even help with his own defense. However, in his rush to dispose of the case, his public defender didn't raise this issue, so I did some digging."

"You did some digging?" I repeat.

"Yep. Got his school records and looked into the background of the other two defendants."

"And what did you find?"

"His school records confirmed my hunch. He'd had an individualized education plan (IEP)[7] because of an intellectual impairment from pre-K through high school. The teachers' comments in his records indicated that he was operating in most academic areas like a fourth or fifth grader. Nonetheless, he was passed on to high school and eventually dropped out at the beginning of 10th grade with no follow up from anyone at the school or the state."

"He had an IEP for an intellectual disability?"

"Yep, and despite it, he fell through the cracks in the system and has been left on his own ever since. If it hadn't had been for his aunt, I don't think he would have survived. She raised him as if he was her son. Got him involved in their local church and kept him from the violence and gangs on the street."

"You said you also looked into the background of his two accomplices?"

Her tone shifts into lawyer mode, which I'm familiar with from Astrid, and I can almost imagine her standing up straight as if she is giving a brief to the court.

"Well, I don't think 'accomplices' is the right term for those two."

"No?"

"Because what I found through my research was that the two other defendants had both been in and out of the legal system for years and had priors for burglary. In fact, they knew each other and had served time for having done the same kind of liquor store robbery together before."

I'm shocked at such an important omission from the record.

"What you're saying is that they set him up?"

----

7. An Individualized Education Program, or IEP, is an educational program tailored to meet the individual needs of students with disabilities.

"Yep!" she exclaims. "And because of the rush to make the plea deal, Claude's version of the story never got in the record."

"Which is what?" I ask, my curiosity elevating.

"That he didn't know the other two men. The first time he'd met them was on the day of the robbery. He'd been working as a day laborer off the books with a group of men from his church on the same construction site they were working on when they approached him. He told me that they seemed nice, and when one of them suggested that after work they go to a local park and drink some beer, he thought they were just being friendly. When he told them he didn't have any money, they both told him that wouldn't be a problem."

My investigator's mind begins to reconstruct the scene: *These two guys, who were planning to rob the liquor store, looked around that construction site for a patsy to take the fall if things went wrong, and here comes Claude, 'a sweet boy, but not too smart', as his aunt put it, walking right into their plan.*

"So, after work, they all go to a liquor store near the construction site. They told him to wait outside. When they came out, they had several bottles of beer and booze, but what Claude did not know was that they also had all the money from the cash register having just robbed the store. Then they all went to a local park where they proceeded to drink, which was where they were arrested several hours later. As planned, they pointed the finger at Claude and got to walk while he took the fall and went to prison for three years."

She's right! This is a travesty of justice! Claude was being set up by these two small-time criminals! This can't get any worse.

"Wait! How did ICE get involved?" I ask, feeling indignant.

"Since 9/11, the prison system routinely advises ICE when they have an undocumented noncitizen in custody. So, when Claude finished his three-year sentence, they met him in the courtyard of the prison, handcuffed him, and took him to the detention center to be processed for deportation.

"When I talked with Claude, it was clear that he had even less understanding about why he was being detained at Valley Forge for the immigration issues than he did about the criminal charges that sent him to prison for three years," she says, her voice now breaking with emotion. "In fact, the man I talked with was confused and frightened. No, terrified! He was terrified, Dr. Gillespie!"

Composing herself, she continues. "And as it turns out, with good reason. A friend of mine from my undergraduate years at Swarthmore who works for the State Department looked into this for me. She agrees with his aunt that based on what they know about the conditions in Haiti, it's unlikely that Claude will survive."

"Ms. Wright, I agree that this sounds like a terrible miscarriage of justice. Actually, it seems tragic to me," I say, feeling moved with compassion over Claude's situation. "The poor guy is getting railroaded, but this seems to be primarily a legal matter, and I'm still unsure what assistance a neuropsychologist like me, or this center, could provide?"

"Dr. Gillespie, I am going to go into the immigration court to block his deportation and into state court to overturn his conviction," she says with resolute determination. "Since Claude's intellectual impairment was never brought up by his public defender, I'm going to assert that he was inadequately represented by his attorney. Specifically, I'm going to appeal his conviction under the 14th Amendment to the Constitution and federal and state statutes arguing that he was denied due process of law because his intellectual impairment prevented him from understanding the nature of the charges against him and assisting in his defense. Additionally, I'm going to argue in immigration court that his deportation would violate the 8th amendment's prohibition again cruel and unusual punishments."

"Wow! And I can help how?" I say, stunned by the audacity of her plan.

"To sustain these arguments, I need to be able to demonstrate that he currently has an intellectual impairment, and to do this, it will require an evaluation. Since Claude has no money, and I don't have the funds to pay for the evaluation, it would have to be pro bono, and I haven't been able to find anyone willing to do it. This is where your clinic comes in. What do you think?"

"Let me get this straight. To save Claude, you are going to bring a legal action against both the federal and state government under the 8th and 14th amendments, and you need a neuropsychological evaluation to do it?"

"Yep."

The malaise I was feeling just moments before evaporates. My admiration for her activism and the audacity of her proposal ignites my passion and makes me want to be a part of it. In some ways, I feel I *need* to be.

"Ms. Wright, by all means, count me in!"

"Pro bono?" she asks.

I cannot think of a better use for my services than to correct an institutional injustice.

"Not a problem," I say. "This is definitely pro bono publico[8]."

Still hesitant, she adds one last detail to our deal.

"There is one more wrinkle to this. Claude is currently in

---

8. Pro Bono Publico, shortened to **pro bono**, is a Latin phrase that means "for the public good" and refers to professional work undertaken voluntarily and without payment.

ICE detention. You would have to travel to Valley Forge to do the evaluation."

Having already committed to the project, I say, "I am sure that my student assistants and I will enjoy the road trip."

"Student assistants?"

"This will be a unique learning opportunity for my neuropsychology grad students to see the potential of these types of assessments in a legal setting. So, while I will be doing the evaluation and signing the report and, if you need, testifying, I would like to bring two of them along as my assistants."

I hear a soft sigh of relief on the phone as she realizes that I'm fully committed.

"That should not be a problem, Doctor. I will send you all my records and when you've had time to review them, get back to me so we can set up a date for the evaluation. I want to be at the facility to introduce you to Claude. He's a bit skittish with strangers after all of this...and thank you."

ICE Moshannon Valley Processing Center
Valley Forge, Pennsylvania, 2006

The woodlands and meadows outside of Philadelphia surround us. As I drive with my two graduate students to the ICE Moshannon Valley Processing Center, Laura[9] a third-year graduate student at the NAC who's close to receiving her doctorate, and Peter[10], a first-year student, nervously sit in the back seat. I selected Laura because she has experience in evaluating intellectual disabilities and Peter because he has a knack

---

9. Name has been changed.
10. Name has been changed.

for picking up details in the evaluation process that often go overlooked.

As we approach the detention center, its tall chain-link fences topped with razor wire and armed guards are enough to intimidate anyone. Glancing at the two students in the back seat, I can see from the stiffness in their postures and the tense expressions on their faces that they are anxious. Even though I briefed them that the evaluation was going to be done off-site, I can see that the oppressive infrastructure is having an effect on them.

Stopping the car about 200 yards from the entrance, I turn and speak to them using the same tone I've used before to lead investigative teams for the government.

"Remember who we are and why we are here. We are neuropsychologists. We represent the university, and we are authorized to be here. Also, what we are going to do here is important."

This seems to calm them a little, but their apprehension still remains palpable.

When I pull up to the gate, the gruff guard asks me for our IDs. I hand them to him, and he looks down to examine each one carefully.

"What is your business here?" he asks with a stern voice.

I can see the students stiffen with anxiety, but I anticipated this and ostentatiously pull out the document that Jacqueline sent me and give it to the guard.

"I'm Dr. Gillespie. I'm a neuropsychologist, and these are my assistants. This is a court order from the chief judge in the immigration court authorizing me to evaluate the individual named in the order who's being detained here. I am to meet with his attorney at the administrative center, and I would appreciate you directing me there."

Startled, the guard looks at the document and then back at

me. When I signal my impatience by beckoning him with my fingers to return the document and our IDs, his attitude quickly changes from ferocious gatekeeper to that of friendly tour guide, and he politely gives me directions to the administrative center. As we drive past the gate, I look at Laura and Peter and see that their anxiety has been replaced by smirking grins. I like to think that they enjoyed my performance.

When we arrive at the administrative center, we notice that this structure is far less intimidating in its design. We park the car and grab our testing equipment before entering the tan brick building. Immediately greeted by a tall, fit woman dressed in a black skirt and suit jacket, my mind immediately identifies that this is Jacqueline Wright. From the way she looks at us, I sense that she's already sized us up and is happy with what she sees.

"Hi, Dr. Gillespie. I'm Jacqueline. It's nice to actually meet you in person."

"Nice to meet you as well. These are Laura and Peter. They will be helping with the evaluation."

"Nice to meet you both."

Jacqueline leads us to a small conference room just off the lobby where the students set up the neuropsychological testing equipment. When we're ready, I give her a thumbs up, and she picks up the phone to make a brief call. A few minutes later, two burly uniformed guards arrive. Their posture dwarfs the unassuming, dark-skinned man wearing an orange jumpsuit who I can only presume is Claude. He hangs his head low, and I notice that he's frightfully thin. Based on the deep circles under his eyes, he hasn't slept in days either.

Claude's eyes dart around the room like a cornered animal. The fear and confusion are clearly discernable and reminds me of the look I saw in Sonny's eyes when he was strapped down in that bed at Anoka, triggering the same intuitive impulse: *I'm not going the leave him here.*

When the guards leave the room, I walk over to Claude to shake his hand.

"Hello, I'm Dr. Gillespie, and I'm here to help you."

Claude hesitates and looks at Jacqueline for reassurance. Only when she nods does he take my hand. He remains silent and avoids eye contact.

Laura, who has seen this type of behavior before with children, intervenes. I watch as she slowly moves toward Claude.

"Hello, Claude. I'm Laura and I have some interesting things for us to do," she says in a bright voice, gently putting her hand on his shoulder.

He looks at her carefully before she escorts him to the table where the neuropsychology testing materials are sprawled out. Breaking the tension, she warms him up by chatting with him about innocuous topics like his favorite food, sports teams, and hobbies. I can see Claude's shoulders drop as he begins to relax.

Claude's evaluation takes a total six hours with each session broken up into two three-hour blocks of testing. We agreed ahead of time that during the morning session, Peter and I would evaluate his cognitive abilities, and that, in the afternoon, Laura would assess his communication and daily living skills as well as his social functioning and emotional coping mechanisms.

At the lunch break, Peter and I have just finished scoring a number of the tests and have a general sense of his IQ and his other cognitive abilities. These include his capacities for attention and concentration, memory, information processing, problem solving, and decision making, all of which will be relevant in determining whether he was able to understand and effectively participate in the legal proceedings.

"His overall functioning falls within the impaired range, but his verbal abilities are much more impaired than his nonverbal ones." I inform Jacqueline. "This means that his ability to do things with his hands is better than his ability to explain or understand things verbally. We also found a wide range of specific neurocognitive deficits with respect to attention, memory, problem-solving, and decision-making."

Jacqueline squints her eyes. "So, that means he *is* intellectually impaired?"

"Short answer, yes. Thus far, the neuropsych data confirms your suspicion of intellectual impairment."

"What will you be doing this afternoon?" she asks, her expression softening.

"This afternoon, Laura will be evaluating how these cognitive deficits affect his social-emotional functioning. This is important in order to demonstrate the real-world implications of these deficits on Claude's day-to-day ability to work, understand things, and take care of himself independently."

We gather again at the end of the day, and Laura connects the dots for Jacqueline.

"His cognitive and social deficits limit his ability to understand complex social situations and render him vulnerable to manipulation by others," she states.

Jacqueline swivels in her chair toward me, speaking in legalese.

"Dr. Gillespie, in your professional opinion as a neuropsychologist and based on your evaluation of the defendant, can you say to any degree of scientific certainty whether he has the requisite intellectual and developmental ability to understand the crime that he was charged with, the legal proceedings, the plea bargain, and his own defense?"

"As a neuropsychologist, it is my professional opinion, based on the results of my direct evaluation of the defendant, that to a degree of scientific certainty because of the cognitive and social developmental deficits he experiences, Claude could not have understood the crime he was charged with or the plea bargain that he was offered. He also could not have meaningfully participated in or assisted his counsel with his defense," I reply, mirroring her legal speak.

"Yes!" she shouts, spontaneously slamming her hand on the conference table.

"It'll take a week or so to finalize the full report, but that's my opinion."

"Great! I'll be in touch," she says as we all file out of the room.

~

Superior Court Appeals
Montgomery County, Pennsylvania, 2007

Sitting uncomfortably on the wooden bench outside the courtroom, I mentally prepare myself to testify. I also can't help but think about the remarkable events that have transpired in the past six months since we first evaluated Claude.

In the interim, Jacqueline has successfully convinced an immigration judge to stay the deportation procedures pending the outcome of her appeals to overturn his conviction in state court. She has also persuaded him, much to our relief, to discharge Claude from the detention center into the care of his aunt. We've also spent countless hours doing careful trial prep with a thoroughness I had not experienced since working as an investigator with the US attorney's office in New York City.

Suddenly, my thoughts are interrupted when one of the tall oak doors to the courtroom opens and a uniformed court officer approaches me.

"Dr. Gillespie, they are ready for you now."

Entering the courtroom, I give Laura and Peter, who are sitting in the gallery as spectators, a furtive smile. When I pass the bar into the well of the room, I see Claude sitting next to Jacqueline. He still looks confused, but he's neatly dressed in a suit that no doubt she provided.

In our trial prep, she told me that based on the appeals judge's questions during the preliminary hearings, the judge is disgusted by the plea-bargaining process that Claude endured.

"Bob, I think he would like to overturn the conviction, but to do that, he needs new evidence that wasn't presented during the initial proceedings. Not to put too much pressure on you, but you are that evidence. I think that the whole case now hinges on the data from the neuropsychological evaluation about the nature and severity of his intellectual impairment. If we can convince him that this proves that Claude didn't and couldn't understand what was going on, then I think he'll overturn it."

Stopping before the witness stand, I raise my right hand, and as I repeat the oath, I experience a nervous sensation in the pit of my stomach similar to when I testified for the government about the accident on the Jersey Turnpike. While I'm confident about my findings, I'm also struck that there are life and death issues at stake. For me, it was an attempted hit; for Claude, it is a virtual death sentence through deportation.

Sitting in the witness stand, Jacqueline begins asking our carefully rehearsed questions. My nerves dissipate as I shift into my role as a neuropsychologist reviewing the data of Claude's examination.

"No further questions, Your Honor," she says, some forty-five minutes later, satisfied she's made her case.

The judge nods to the state prosecutor who rises to begin his cross examination.

Unlike with therapy where the focus is to help someone, the courtroom is an adversarial arena in which winning is the main objective. The goal of the cross-examination is to undermine the validity of the assessment and my credibility with a set of carefully worded questions.

The example I use with my graduate students is the classic question taught in law classes: *Have you stopped beating your wife? Yes or no?*

Lawyers love these types of questions because no matter how the defendant answers, by default, the implication is that either the beatings have occurred or are still occurring.

While I'm quite comfortable discussing the scientific facts of Claude's condition, the intensity of the cross-examination is more heightened than usual because the state prosecutor who had Claude thrown in jail for three years is irate that Jacqueline's trying to move this case from his win column to his loss column. He knows that he can't argue the facts, only my opinion.

Lawyers typically question an expert's credentials and/or the science behind their findings. Since Jacqueline has already established my credentials as a neuropsychologist, the first avenue of his attack is blocked. His only choice is to undermine the nature of the evaluation and the science behind our conclusions regarding Claude's mental state.

While straightening his suit jacket, the prosecutor directs his attention to me.

"Dr. Gillespie, could you walk me in detail through the neuropsychological evaluation process you used to make your determination?"

I describe the tests that were used, who administered them, and the setting in which it was completed. Looking for a weakness in the testing process, the lawyer focuses on who administered the exam—my students.

"So, some of the tests were administered by graduate students who are not licensed psychologists? Is that right?"

"Yes. Each of them has been extensively trained by me and other neuropsychologists at the center with respect to the specific tests they administered, and, in my professional judgement, were qualified to do so. Also, I was physically in the room observing them as they performed these tests. It's a common practice in my profession to use assistants in this manner as long as there's an expert present to supervise and observe them. However, the opinions expressed in this report are based on my professional judgement, not theirs."

Feeling that he'd reached a dead end, he shifts to another line of attack.

"Well, then let's explore the data that you based your opinion on, shall we? First of all, can you explain to me why you chose the specific tests that were used?"

Suspecting that this might be a trick question, I respond choosing my words carefully.

"The battery of tests I used is considered to be the standard test protocol for this type of evaluation in the psychological and medical community."

He allows me to detail the specific reasons and uses for each test, hoping that I'll stumble.

Unable to find a weakness, he tries to exploit the scientific validity of the social-emotional evaluation Laura administered. However, having spent three years teaching courses to doctoral students on the science behind the neuropsychological instruments we use in our evaluations, including the ones Laura used to evaluate Claude, I'm quite comfortable discussing their scientific reliability.

"So, based on your evaluation, you determined that your client had a severe intellectual impairment, right?"

Sensing a set up, I answer tersely, "Yes."

He then springs the lawyer's question.

"Yes or no, Dr. Gillespie. Isn't it possible that someone with this level of intellectual impairment would steal something?" he asks smugly.

Suddenly, I recall an important piece of advice given to me by an assistant U.S. attorney. As a young investigator headed to court to give sworn testimony for the first time, he said, "Remember, on cross-examination, only answer the question being asked. Don't elaborate."

This is generally good advice, but I'm about to break that rule.

"Of course, it's possible, but in Claude's case—"

"Objection! Your Honor, the witness is being nonresponsive. That is beyond the scope of my question. I did not ask about his client."

With the trap sprung, the prosecutor is implying that Claude had the capacity to rob the liquor store, suggesting that his intellectual impairment is an insufficient basis to overturn the conviction.

This is a difficult situation. Answering with a simple 'no' is not going to work since it's technically incorrect. Someone with Claude's impairments *could* steal, but in his case, it isn't true. He was the patsy to someone else's crime. However, answering with a simple 'yes' without qualifying the answer would grant the prosecutor's point.

The court room falls silent. All eyes are on the judge as we wait for him to either sustain or overrule the objection. I feel the heavy weight of anxiety bearing down on me as I look out at the courtroom and see Jacqueline sitting ramrod straight with her gaze laser focused on the judge. Laura and Peter are seated in the back, holding their breath.

After a few moments, the judge addresses the prosecutor.

"Overruled, counselor. I would be very interested to hear what Dr. Gillespie has to say."

I hear an audible but delighted gasp from Laura and Peter.

"Order in the court! There will be no outbursts!" shouts the judge, slamming his gavel against the sounding block. "Please, continue, Doctor."

"Thank you, Your Honor. What I was about to say was that while it's true that an intellectual impairment does not preclude someone from engaging in bad behavior, in Claude's case, his level of development and social history actually does. From our evaluation, it's clear that he has a concrete level of moral development in which things are black or white—either right or wrong. For him, stealing is among the things that are wrong. Developmentally, he is similar to a typical fourth grader, and for individuals at this stage of development, there are no gray areas."

The judge interrupts. "Doctor, how does that bear on the prosecutor's question?"

"I was just getting to that, Your Honor. Up to the point of the liquor store incident, Claude had no prior criminal record of any type. There is no history of stealing or shop lifting, and his school records did not indicate any behavioral problems. Interpersonally, he is passive and shy and, because of his cognitive limitations, naïve and easily manipulated. This is simply not the profile of someone who suddenly decides to rob a liquor store. Nor, as he was accused of, is he someone with the capacity to plan and execute such a robbery, which brings me to my final point."

Pausing for effect I look around the courtroom. The prosecutor is fuming. Jacqueline and the judge are intensely focused on me.

"In the original investigation, it was alleged by the other defendants, who each had a history of planning and committing similar burglaries, that the idea to rob the liquor store was Claude's. Based on the data from our evaluation, it is my professional opinion to a degree of scientific certainty that given Claude's intellectual limitations, it would not have been possible for him to have planned the robbery. While Claude can follow simple instructions and engage in routine and repetitive behaviors, he does not have the intellectual ability to plan and independently initiate complex behavior. Combining this with his social and developmental limitations, it would not have been possible for him to have convinced the others to commit the robbery nor carry it out. Also, while he is vulnerable to the exploitation of others for their own self-interest, seeing that it as a wrongful act, our data indicates that he would not have knowingly agreed to be a part of such an activity."

Keeping my attention focused on the judge, I take a deep breath before continuing.

"And, Your Honor, because of these same severe limitations, he also could not have understood what he was being charged with or be able to have meaningfully assisted his counsel in his own defense," I say, adding the final nail to the coffin.

The judge gives me a knowing—and almost imperceptible—nod.

"Thank you, Doctor. Does counsel have any further questions?"

"No further questions, Your Honor," the prosecutor says, slumping down in his chair.

The judge dismisses me from the courtroom, and I wait outside accompanied by Laura and Peter.

Two grueling hours later, a jubilant Jacqueline bursts through the courtroom doors and hugs me.

"We won! He overturned it!" she shouts. "He didn't even

delay and take it under advisement. He said Claude should never have been tried in the first place, threw out the plea agreement and dismissed the original charges in the interest of justice. Claude's been exonerated! His aunt is beside herself with joy, and I'm pretty sure I saw Claude smile even though I don't think he fully understood what happened! Thank you!"

"No. Thank *you,* Jacqueline. We are proud to have been involved in Claude's case, and it's been a privilege to work with someone like you."

The tension we all felt since this case began turns into a burst of emotional exuberance. Everybody hugs and high fives each other. Turning to Laura and Peter, whose eyes are glowing with pride, I grin and say, "And that's the kind of neuropsychology I like to practice!"

~

Neuropsychology Assessment Center
Chester, Pennsylvania, 2008

While the successful outcome of Claude's case was an incredible experience for everyone involved, it alleviated my professional restlessness only briefly. I still find myself haunted by the image of Claude as he entered the testing room standing between those two guards—an image that highlights the continued abuse and exploitation of people with disabilities. It's a need that I saw at the Institute and the NBI but was unable to address in my current role as a director of a university-based training clinic.

These thoughts continue to percolate over the next few months, gathering momentum as I consider whether I should leave the NAC—a decision that's complicated by the impact it would have on my family. Astrid is happy at her job with the

Inquirer; my youngest son is about to graduate from high school and move to college, and my eldest is doing a year of community service with AmeriCorps in Philadelphia. Also, there are perks and enticements to remaining in an academic setting and conducting research, so I dither for a few weeks.

That is, until I receive a letter from Jacqueline Wright that awakens my true passion.

Dear Dr. Gillespie,

I want to again thank you, your students, and the Neuropsychology Assessment Center for the work you did on Claude's behalf. I also want to bring you up to date on what has happened to him. After the trial, I got in contact with the Department of Human Services and the Office of Developmental Programs. After some administrative wrangling, I was able to get him enrolled in a vocational training program. He is now learning carpentry. He still lives with his aunt, but he has made friends with several of the other trainees. It sounds like they may all move in together after they complete their training and get jobs. However, what I'm most excited about is that I've found an advocacy group that works with Haitian immigrants, and they are working with Claude on his becoming a citizen. I'm also now very busy with similar appeals cases in my legal aid practice, but I intend to continue keeping an eye on Claude's development.

You may not realize it, but the evaluation that you and your team did saved Claude's life, and we are both very grateful. Thank you.

Sincerely,

Jacquie

Jacqueline S. Wright, J.D.
Attorney at Law

Re-reading her letter causes the shadows of uncertainty to lift. I come to a realization about how I can best practice neuropsychology.

In my career, I've enjoyed building and administering clinical programs like NBI and NAC and doing research, but what has truly given me a sense of professional fulfillment and satisfaction is using what I've learned to directly help my patients. Even though I left the agency three decades ago, I'm still most comfortable thinking and acting like a government investigator working the streets, collecting data, and trying to uncover the patterns of human behavior—all of which makes the laurels of academia and the prestige of a corporate suite a poor fit for me. They're too remote. Too far off from the patients I'm meant to serve. They're not gritty enough for the kind of clinical work I have in mind. To do what I want, I need to be in the field again closer to those I serve.

Folding the letter, I place it inside my jacket pocket over my heart. I've come to a decision. My work at Widener and the NAC is complete. It's time to leave the ivory-towers of academia and re-enter the world of clinical practice. Now is the time to find new collaborators and adventurers who are willing to explore the uncharted archipelago of the human mind in search of our *shared humanity*. After all, we humans have more in common with the least of us—even the worst of us—than any other living thing on the planet.

Until next time...

Questions for Consideration

1. What were the shortfalls in Claude's case the first time he went to court? How did Jacqueline find out about the case? Why do you think she selected it? Also, why did she choose the author to work with her? How did she know that he would be able to help Claude?

2. How did the author prepare for the case? How do you think that his investigative instincts helped navigate this particular event? Do you think that the author felt a sense of satisfaction or relief when the case was over? Which emotion do you think the students felt?

3. How did the author prepare the students for future leadership roles, especially in how he presented the evidence for this case? What do you think that they learned from this case that they could take with them into their own careers? What potential did the author see in them? Why do you think they were handpicked for this? After the author chose them, what did he do to support them and mentor them?

4. Do you think that the students conducting the tests enabled the author to make observations that he would have missed if he were doing it himself?

5. How did Claude's lack of education and ability to comprehend his situation affect him? How did this case impact his future and his potential to live in the United States? What role did Claude's disability play in his not receiving an equitable education or legal treatment? Why did Claude's lawyer not represent him? What did his lawyer have to gain, or do you believe that he was just drawing a paycheck because he was court appointed? Do you think that

the lawyer simply didn't care because Claude had a disability?

6. What kind of resources would you personally set up for Claude if you were his attorney? What things are most important to you when working with this clinical population? What would have been most important to Claude? How would you have found out about his interests and abilities?

7. What do you think was the first thing Claude wanted to do when he got out of prison?

8. Claude's aunt said he wasn't "too smart." Why do you think that she chose to frame his learning disability in this manner? Do you think that Claude's lawyer took advantage of that comment? Do you think that the aunt felt that Claude would be better off in prison so that he would be taken care of? Could she have seen him as a burden?

BIBLIOGRAPHY

Cooney, N., Gillespie, R., Baker, L., Kaplan, R. 1987. "Cognitive Changes After Alcohol Cue Exposure." *Journal of Consulting and Clinical Psychology.* (55): 150-155.

Exner, J., Viglione, D., Gillespie, R. 1984. "Relationships between Rorschach variables as relevant to the interpretation of structural data." *Journal of Personality Assessment.*, (48): 65-70.

Eysenck, H. J. 1952. "The effects of psychotherapy: an evaluation." *Journal of Consulting Psychology, 16* (5): 319-324

Frances, A. "Mislabeling Medical Illness as Mental Disorder." *Psychology Today* (blog). December 8, 2012,
https://www.psychologytoday.com/us/blog/dsm5-in-distress/201212/mislabel ing-medical-illness-mental-disorder

Frankl, V.E. 1963. *Man's Search for Meaning: An Introduction to Logotherapy.* Washington Square Press.

Freud, S. 1961. *The Ego and the Id.* W. W. Norton & Co.

Freud, S. 1949. *An Outline of Psychoanalysis.* W. W. Norton & Co.

Freud, S. 1933. *New Introductory Lectures on Psychoanalysis.* Norton & Co.

Freud, S., & Breuer, J. 1895. *Studies on Hysteria.* (Translated by James Strachey, 1955). Basic Books.

Gillespie, R. 1986. "Relapse and Conditioning: Cognitive and Physiological Changes in Alcoholics After Exposure to Alcohol." (Ph.D. diss., Long Island University) Dissertation Abstracts International. 46:2806B.

Gillespie, R. 2013. *Diagnostic and Statistical Manual of Mental Disorders* (5th ed.; DSM-5). American Psychiatric Association.

BIBLIOGRAPHY

Gillespie, R. & Gillespie, R. 2021. *Journeys of the Heart.* Unpublished Song/Poem

Gillespie, R. 2021. *Transcendence.* Unpublished Song/Poem

Gillespie, R., Ormiston, C., Sarff, P. June, 1994. "Analysis of Treatment Outcomes for Brain Injured Patients in Intensive Inpatient Neurobehavioral Treatment." *American Society of Neurorehabilitation.*

Gottesman, I. I. 1991. *Schizophrenia Genesis: The Origins of Madness.* W H Freeman/Times Books/ Henry Holt & Co.

Higley, B.M. 1873. *My Western Home.* The Smith County Pioneer.

Kaplan, R., Cooney, N., Baker, L., Gillespie, R., Meyer, R., Pomerleau, O. 1985. "Reactivity to Alcohol-Related Cues: Physiological and Subjective Responses in Alcoholics and Non-Problem Drinkers." *Journal of Studies on Alcohol.* (46): 276-272.

Kendler, K. S., et al. 1993. "The Genetic Epidemiology of Schizophrenia." *Journal of the American Medical Association.*

King, S. 1978. *The Stand.* Doubleday

Kuhn, T. S. 1962. *The Structure of Scientific Revolutions.* University of Chicago Press.

Laing, R.D. 1967. *The Politics of Experience.* Ballantine Books

Lamott, A 2008. *Grace (Eventually): Thoughts on Faith.* Penguin

Lazarus, E. 1883. *Statue of Liberty* [Inscription].

Selye H. 1946. "The General Adaptation Syndrome and the Diseases of Adaptation." *Journal of Clinical Endocrinology* (6):117-231

Seltzberg, H., Ehrie, J. & Goldwaser, E. 2024. "Genetics and Schizophrenia." *Curr Behav Neurosci Rep* (11): 57-63 https://doi.org/10.1007/s40473-024-00274-x

Singh, H. 2018. "Suicide in Schizophrenia Spectrum Disorders: A Review of

Socio-Demographic and Clinical Correlates." *Indian Journal of Private Psychiatry* 12 (1): 20-26 DOI:10.5005/jp-journals-10067-0013.

Sullivan, H. S. 1954. *The Psychiatric Interview.* W. W. Norton & Co.

Sullivan, H. S. 1953. *The Interpersonal Theory of Psychiatry.* W W Norton & Co.

Tolkien, J. R. R. 1991. *The Fellowship of the Ring.* HarperCollins

Viereck, G.S. October 26, 1929. "What Life Means to Einstein: An Interview". *Saturday Evening Post.*

Wilde, O., & Holloway, J. 1911. *Lady Windermere's Fan: A Play About a Good Woman* (Sixth Edition). Methuen.

Wilder, Thornton. 1938. *Our Town: A Play in Three Acts.* Published by Harper & Row, 1985.

Yalom, I. D. 1995. *The Theory and Practice of Group Psychotherapy* (4th ed.). Basic Books